Breath of Life

The Role of the Ventilator in Managing Life-Threatening Illnesses

Irene S. Gilgoff
and the
Editors of the American Institute of Life-Threatening Illness and Loss

The Scarecrow Press, Inc.
Lanham, Maryland, and London
2002

SCARECROW PRESS, INC.

Published in the United States of America
by Scarecrow Press, Inc.
4720 Boston Way, Lanham, Maryland 20706
www.scarecrowpress.com

4 Pleydell Gardens, Folkestone
Kent CT20 2DN, England

British Library Cataloguing-in-Publication Information Available

Library of Congress Cataloging-in-Publication Data

Gilgoff, Irene S.
Breath of life : the role of the ventilator in managing life-threatening illnesses / Irene S. Gilgoff and the editors of the American Institute of Life-Threatening Illness and Loss.
p. cm.
Includes bibliographical references.
ISBN 0-8108-3488-X (alk. paper)
1. Respiratory therapy. 2. Artificial respiration. 3. Respirators (Medical equipment) I. American Institute of Life-Threatening Illness and Loss. II. Title.
[DNLM: 1. Respiration, Artificial—psychology. 2. Ventilators, Mechanical. 3. Informed Consent. 4. Life Support Care. 5. Medical Futility. 6. Patient Advocacy. WF 26 G473b 2001]
RM161.G55 2002
615.8'36—dc21 2001020287

™ The paper used in this publication meets the minimum requirements of American National Standard for Information Sciences—Permanence of Paper for Printed Library Materials, ANSI/NISO Z39.48-1992.
Manufactured in the United States of America.

CONTENTS

ACKNOWLEDGMENT

The authors wish to express appreciation for the support and encouragement of The American Institute of Life-Threatening Illness and Loss, a division of The Foundation of Thanatology, in the preparation of this volume. Thanatology, a new subspecialty of medicine, is involved in scientific and humanistic inquiries and the application of the knowledge derived therefrom to the subjects of the medical and psychological aspects of life-threatening illness.

The American Institute is dedicated to advancing the cause of enlightened health care for the life-threatened patient and his or her family. The Institute's orientation is a positive one based on the philosophy of fostering a more mature acceptance and understanding of serious illness and the problems involved.

LIST OF CONTRIBUTORS

Augusta Alba
Shirley M. Acosta
Albert Anderson
John R. Bach
Margaret E. Backman
Rana A. Bahl
Ahmet Baydur
Barbara T. Beal
James C. Bernier
Ann Burkhardt
Agatha P. Colbert
Barbara J. Daly
Pamela K. Dewitt
Karen Dikeman
Kathleen J. Dunleavy
Esther Ehrenberg
Jack Genskow
Irene S. Gilgoff
Sarah J. Gossler
Daniel Heilburn
Ira W. Holland
Frank T. Hsieh
Guo-Long Hung
Mary T. Jansen
Emily Kahlstrom
Paul Kahn
Joseph Kaufert
Marta Kazandjian
Susan E. Keens
Thomas G. Keens
Audrey J. King
Terry Kinzel
Sckhar C. Kota
Gini Laurie
Eric M. Levander
Lee E. Lipsker
David Locker
Eithne MacLaughlin
Julie G. Madorsky
Bente Madsen
Frederick M. Maynard
Margaret Mikol
Masakuni Mukoyama
Syed Ejaz Naqvi
Hugh Newton-John
Edward Anthony Oppenheimer
Marilyn M. Rawnsley
Radha J. Sarma
Charles A. Stewart
Robert Sudrann
Sally L. Davidson Ward
Jon E. Woo

1

A REVIEW OF VENTILATOR USE IN DUCHENNE'S MUSCULAR DYSTROPHY

Agatha P. Colbert, M.D.

The use of assisted ventilation by individuals with Duchenne's muscular dystrophy (DMD) has been in effect for the past 25 to 30 years. As in other management issues for DMD (i.e., lower extremity soft tissue surgery, with or without the use of orthotics; a physical therapy program of stretching or strengthening; and surgical stabilization of the spine), there is, and probably will continue to be, recurrent debate regarding the cost/benefit ratio of various treatment regimens. I come to this issue from an emotional, pyschosocial, and ethical perspective, as well as a financial point of view.

The decision to ventilate, and which ventilator to employ, is frequently made for the individual patient and his or her family by the attending physician, according to his or her own personal experience and philosophical orientation. In a 1985 survey, 44 percent of the Muscular Dystrophy Association Clinic directors said they routinely provided respiratory support systems to people with certain specific diseases, while 24 percent never prescribed them (Colbert, 1985). The remaining clinicians offered assisted ventilation to certain patients in select situations.

Some medical centers advocate tracheotomies with positive pressure ventilators (Baydur, 1990), while others maintain that mouth intermittent positive pressure systems are the best means of assisting ventilation (Bach, 1987). More recently, nasal mask-assisted ventilation has been increasingly favored (Bach, 1990; Ellis, 1987; Kerby, 1987; Segall, 1988). Still other clinicians report success with negative pressure body ventilators (Curran, 1989).

It is not the ambition of this chapter to resolve this debate. The technological aids for ventilating with DMD are readily available in the United States and have been proven effective for those using them. As long as we as a society have the funding to supply kidney, liver, bone marrow, and heart and lung transplants to people needing them, it is difficult to accept the argument that a ventilator, which is significantly less costly, should not be offered to someone with chronic respiratory failure desirous of prolonging his or her life (Plough, 1986).

The decision belongs to the individual and his or her family, who must live with the aftermath of their choice. The role of health care professionals is to collect and disseminate as much data as possible regarding types of ventilators, further medical complications in DMD, and daily quality of life issues, so that those most intimately involved can make an adequately informed decision.

The results of some extraordinarily successful research into the cause and possible treatments for DMD have been published. The locus of the gene for DMD on the long arm of the X chromosome was defined. Shortly thereafter, the missing protein, dystrophin, was identified (Hoffman, 1988). The potential for treatment to "cure" or halt the progression of the disease may actually be in sight with myoblast transfers and gene therapy (Law, 1988; Wolff, 1990). These recent breakthroughs encourage a more optimistic approach with regard to the preservation of life and function in individuals with DMD.

A brief review of the natural history of DMD reads as follows: children are diagnosed with the disease between the ages of two and five years. They experience difficulty with ambulation by age nine or ten, and although lower extremity bracing with or without surgery may prolong walking another two years, all patients are wheelchair users by age 12. Scoliosis begins shortly thereafter and progresses rapidly and to a significant degree by the age of 16 (Colbert, 1987; Lord, 1990). The combination of a severely deformed spine and respiratory compromise necessitates provision of an appropriately supportive motorized wheelchair if the person is to remain mobile and not become bedridden (Colbert, 1985). Death occurs on the average at 19 years if the disease is allowed to take its natural course.

Approximately 90 percent of deaths from DMD are the result of chronic respiratory failure and/or concurrent respiratory infection. Another 5 to 10 percent die from cardiac causes (Gilroy, 1963). Respiratory failure in neuromuscular diseases is of the restrictive type, resulting from progressive weakness of the muscles of breathing. Intrinsic lung tissue remains intact. As a consequence, the ventilator simply replaces or augments the failed bellows mechanism of the respiratory system.

Several pioneers in this field have advocated and implemented the use of assisted ventilation in the Duchenne population. The first publication to address the matter described three patients who used a variety of noninvasive ventilatory techniques (Aberion, 1973). The devices had been developed during the era of acute polio epidemics, and found ready application in persons with progressive neuromuscular disease. Hill (1986) provided a comprehensive survey of the body ventilators most frequently used. These include the iron lung, porta lung, pneumo wrap, chest shell, pneumo belt, rocking bed, and nose or mouth positive pressure masks.

The Ohio State group reported on ten patients living at home and using similar devices (Alexander, et al., 1979). It was pointed out that life could be prolonged successfully with a ventilator and that the quality of that life was "good," with no need for an invasive procedure such as a tracheotomy.

Curran (1981) published the first systematic study on the long-term effects of negative pressure ventilation, showing that nine patients with DMD could be sustained for several years on nighttime ventilation alone. He applied the principle of respiratory muscle sparing demonstated by Rochester and Braun (1977) in patients with chronic chest wall restriction. By allowing complete rest of the respiratory muscles at night, these young men could be up in wheelchairs, ventilator free, during the daytime, while maintaining normal arterial blood gases.

In the same year, Bach (1981) published a series of 29 patients with progressive muscular dystrophy. Ten were able to use noninvasive ventilatory devices for an average of six years prior to requiring a tracheotomy.

Although there are many accounts of ventilator use among polio survivors in other parts of the world, most of the publications documenting experiences of people with DMD using ventilators have come from the United States. One notable exception is the comprehensive work of Rideau (1981) in France, who performed a longitudinal study of pulmonary function in 90 patients with DMD. He was able to categorize them according to the peak vital capacity reached. Measurements of forced vital capacity (FVC) in each patient revealed a rising phase, a plateau, and a declining phase. On the basis of these groupings, clinicians can better predict the rate of progression of the disease and anticipate when assisted ventilation will be needed. He published his own series of studies of ten boys who received tracheotomies and used positive pressure ventilators (1983), emphasizing the portability of this type of system. He did report, however, that two catastrophic events occurred. One patient died when his tracheotomy tube slipped out, unnoticed, and the other when the tube eroded into the aorta, causing a massive hemorrhage. These two case scenarios serve as a reminder of the potential risks associated with tracheotomy (an invasive procedure) and the need for 24-hour surveillance when the subject is completely dependent on artificial life support.

Our own clinical experience at Lakeville Hospital and New England Medical Center has, until these past three years, been almost exclusively with negative pressure body ventilators in the DMD population. Several circumstances have influenced our decision to employ this type of devices: they have been readily available at our hospital; we have been concerned about the potential complications of a tracheotomy; and in the state of Massachusetts it has been very difficult to place a child in the public school system if he is using a trachestomy with a positive pressure ventilator. For children and young adults with DMD, school provides the main opportunity for socialization, and quality of life diminishes considerably if this activity is precluded.

The effectiveness of nose or mouth intermittent positive pressure ventilation is presently being studied (Bach, 1987; Rideau, 1983; Segall, 1988). The results look promising with regard to preventing the microatelectasis which occurs during sleep and in terms of correcting nocturnal hypoxemia.

Assessing quality of life for individuals with late stage DMD who are ventilator dependent has been a major consideration for health care professionals involved in the care of severely disabled people (Gilgoff, 1981; Robins Miller, 1988). Gilgoff looked specifically at this area in her initial publication on five young men from Rancho Los Amigos, all of whom had tracheotomies and used positive pressure devices. She found that quality of life for these patients did not change significantly with the addition of ventilatory equipment. They remained mobile in power wheelchairs and several described sleeping better and feeling more energetic after initiating ventilator use. Robins Miller has since completed a more extensive study of ventilator users and compared quality of life for those living at home with those residing in institutional settings. Her findings are reported in another chapter of this text.

As more and more individuals with DMD are being ventilated and living an additional 5, 10, or 15 years beyond the expected period of survival, other considerations arise. Doctor Curran and myself (1989) published a 12-year follow up of 23 patients who used primarily noninvasive forms of ventilation. We reported six deaths. Three patients had gone on to elective tracheotomies. The information derived from that study correlates with others (Bach, 1987; Baydur, 1990). Chronic respiratory failure (CRF) occurs at an average age of 19 years 9 months in DMD. The average vital capacity at the onset of symptoms of CRF is 500 mls or 13 percent of the predicted. The most common symptoms of CRF in this group are those consistent with carbon dioxide retention, i.e., morning headache, sleeplessness at night requiring frequent turning, daytime fatigue, weight loss, and depression.

The patients in the study had to increase their time on the ventilator an average of one hour per year per patient. The FVC drops more slowly after initiation of assisted ventilation, but continues to decline. Since the study was published, six additional patients have undergone elective tracheotomies and there have been four more deaths. One patient died the day after his tracheotomy from his severe cardiomyopathy. Another expired one month later, probably as a result of a cardiac arrhythmia. A third died a year later when his tracheotomy tube slipped out and the ventilator alarm system failed. The fourth, who had not received a tracheotomy, died after a month-long hospitalization from an illness of unclear etiology.

In addition to the increased mortality in the patients with advanced DMD, we have seen several complications involving the smooth muscle in the gastrointestinal tract and the genitourinary tract. Five patients developed difficulty swallowing and now require a permanent gastrostomy tube. One developed acute gastric dilatation and four others a pseudo-obstruction of the bowel. Two patients developed acute urinary retention associated with receiving the antidepressant drug Amitryptylline, and one of these had hydroureters with evidence of pseudo-obstruction on intravenous pyelogram. Another of the patients who had had a tracheotomy had significant problems with hypothermia and an inability to maintain core body temperature above 94 degrees Centigrade without external sources of heat.

All patients temporarily lost the ability to speak after the tracheotomy procedure, but subsequently regained the ability as a result of deflating the cuff on the tracheotomy tube and allowing a leak of air to pass up through the vocal cords on inspiration. The presence of the leak necessitated an increase in the volume of air delivered by the ventilator.

A word on cardiac involvement is appropriate. It is well known that patients with DMD have a cardiomyopathy with classical EKG findings (D'Orsagni, 1988). A small minority, however, become symptomatic. Contrary to the findings of Hunsaker (1982), our clinical experience and the work of Stewart and Gilgoff (1988) did not find a correlation between the degree of musculoskeletal deterioration and cardiac dysfunction. Skeletal muscle loss does correlate with decline in pulmonary function, but does not seem to be related to the degree of cardiac fibrosis. We have witnessed five patients dying of severe congestive cardiac failure several years before respiratory failure was anticipated, i.e., FVC was well above 2000 mls. As a corollary, we also have 12 patients who have been ventilator dependent for more than six years, whose left ventricular ejection fractions on echocardiogram remain above 40 percent.

It is apparent from the literature that the techniques for providing assisted ventilation in DMD patients vary considerably in the US and Europe, according to what devices are available and the preference of the prescribing physician. It is also evident that a wide variety of modalities can provide effective treatment to a large number of patients for a long time.

Reflecting on our experience with body ventilators, we realize that all patients with DMD will eventually become 24-hour dependent on a ventilator. As a consequence we are questioning our protocol of prescribing noninvasive systems for the first few years. Can these individuals be adequately sustained on mouth or nose intermittent positive pressure, as suggested by Bach (1987, 1990)? We have not found success with this practice in our clinic as yet. Would it be preferable to proceed immediately to tracheotomy, as is the practice of Rideau and Gilgoff? Certainly the surgical procedure has associated risks. Is it better to perform a tracheotomy when the patient is of "healthier constitution"? Or, if a tracheotomy is delayed, for how long: when the person is dependent 12 hours? 14 hours?

16 hours? Some of our patients who had a tracheotomy after more than seven years on a ventilator became dependent immediately on positive pressure machines for 24 hours a day. Prior to the insertion of the tracheotomy, they had been able to use glossopharyngeal breathing to supplement respiration during the six to eight hours of freedom from the ventilator. The sudden recognition of being totally dependent on a life support system was a source of great distress to two patients, leading to anxiety, sleeplessness, and several months of depression.

Until we have answers to these questions, our current modus operandi is to provide the individual and his or her family with as much information as possible prior to the onset of respiratory failure. This includes all the data on long-term medical complications and quality of life issues that we have gathered over the past 12 years. We introduce them to other ventilator-assisted patients with DMD; we refer those in the process of deciding whether to use a ventilator to a counselor who can assist them in defining the elements of quality of life which are important to them and help assess the impact that the various types of ventilators may have on that quality of life. Finally, we allow each patient to make his or her own decision. We then try to accommodate with the ventilator of choice, if the decision is to prolong life. If the choice is to allow the disease to take its natural course, we try to assist the patient in a peaceful and dignified death. The latter path has been somewhat more difficult for us, as our natural inclination has been to extend what *we* see as a reasonably good quality of life, despite disability.

I would like to conclude with a passage from a letter sent to me by the mother of a 17-year-old with DMD who had to endure the consequences of a lack of communication between the medical staff and the family. She, her husband, and their son had made the decision not to use mechanical ventilation and to keep him home during the terminal stage of the disease. On the day of his death, he was brought to the chronic care hospital precisely because, as his mother later told us, there was no emergency room at our facility! Although she and her husband had reflected deeply on the quality of life and death they wished for their son, this message had not come across to the MDA staff. As a consequence, they brought him to the hospital with the expectation of receiving comfort in his final hours. The hospital personnel, unaware of the family's wishes, interpreted this 8:00 A.M. "emergency visit" to the hospital as an expression of the desire to institute life saving measures. The results were frustrating to both nurses and doctors, as well as an unnecessary crisis for the family.

> *We chose never to have J in a iron lung. He never wanted it and neither did we. In his final twenty minutes of life, the hospital took over and still tried the lung—so futile and so unnecessary. J was dying and the fighting was over. Why couldn't they give him oxygen or just let nature do its work? Parents are in no shape at that point to continue their fight for a rightful*

ending. Why do hospitals still play their roles in these most unique patients—save a life, no matter how futile, no matter how invasive, no matter how devastating. It's frightful and so unnecessary. It could have been so much kinder and we are left with an unforgettable memory of our son's death after we had worked so hard to give him the best life possible. It didn't have to be that way.

Indeed it didn't have to be that way. We health care professionals continue to have much to learn from the experiences and the wisdom of our patients and their families.

REFERENCES

Aberion, G., A. Alba, M.H.M. Solomon, and M.Lee, "Pulmonary Care of Duchenne-type Muscular Dystrophy," *New York J Med*, 1973;15:1206–1207.

Alexander, M.A., E.W. Johnson, J. Petty, and D. Stauch, "Mechanical Ventilation of Patients with Late Stage Duchenne Muscular Dystrophy: Management in the Home," *Arch Phys Med Rehabil*, 1979;60:289–92.

Bach, J.R., and A.S. Alba, "Management of Chronic Alveolar Hypoventilation by Nasal Ventilation," *Chest*, 1990;97:52–57.

Bach, J.R., J. O'Brien, R. Krotenberg, and A.S. Alba, "Management of the End Stage Respiratory Failure in Duchenne Muscular Dystrophy," *Muscle Nerve*, 1987;10:177–182.

Bach J., A. Alba, L.A. Pilkington, and M. Lee, "Long-term Rehabilitation in Advanced Stage of Childhood Onset, Rapidly Progressive Muscular Dystrophy," *Arch Phys Med Rehabil*, 1981;62:328–31.

Baydur, A., I. Gilgoff, W. Prentice, M. Carlson, and D.A. Fisher, "Decline in Respiratory Function and Experience with Long-term Assisted Ventilation in Advanced Duchenne's Muscular Dystrophy," *Chest*, 1990;97:884–89.

Colbert, A.P., and C. Craig, "Scoliosis Management in Duchenne Muscular Dystrophy," *Arch Phys Med Rehabil*, 1987;68:302–304.

Colbert, A.P., and N.A. Schock, "Respirator Use in Progressive Neuromuscular Diseases," *Arch Phys Med Rehabil*, 1985;66:760–762.

Colbert, A.P., J.A. Freyermuth, and F.J. Curran, "Seating and Mobility for Advanced Stage Duchenne Muscular Dystrophy," *Arch Phys Med Rehabil* (Abstr), 1985;66:530.

Curran, F.J., "Night Ventilation by Body Respirators for Patients in Chronic Respiratory Failure Due to Late Stage Duchenne Muscular Dystrophy," *Arch Phys Med Rehabil,* 1981;62:328–31.

Curran, F.J., and A.P. Colbert, "Ventilator Management in Duchenne Muscular Dystrophy and Postpoliomyelitis Syndrome: Twelve Years Experience," *Arch Phys Med Rehabil,* 1989:70:180–185.

D'Orsagni, L., J.P. O'Shea, and G. Miller, "Cardiomyopathy of Duchenne Muscular Dystrophy," *Pediatr Cardiol,* 1988;9:205–213.

Ellis, E.R., et al., "Treatment of Respiratory Failure During Sleep in Patients with Neuromuscular Disease: Positive Pressure Ventilation though a Nose Mask," *Am Rev Respir Dis,* 1987;135:148–152.

Gilgoff, I.S., "End Stage Duchenne Patients: Choosing between Respirator and Natural Death," in L.I. Charash et al., eds., *Psychosocial Aspects of Muscular Dystrophy and Allied Diseases* (Springfield, IL: Charles C. Thomas, 1981).

Gilroy J., J.L. Cahalan, R. Berman, and R. Newman, "Cardiac and Pulmonary Complications in Duchenne's Progressive Muscular Dystrophy," *Circulation,* 1963;27:484–93.

Hill, N.S., "Clinical Applications of Body Ventilators," *Chest,* 1986;90:897–905.

Hoffman, E.P., et al., "Characterization of Dystrophin in Muscle-biopsy Specimens from Patients with Duchenne's or Becker's Muscular Dystrophy," *N Engl J Med,* 1988;318:1363–1368.

Hunsaker, R.H., P.K. Fulkerson, F.J. Barry, et al., "Cardiac Function in Duchenne's Muscular Dystrophy: Results of 10 Year Follow-up Study and Noninvasive Tests," *Am J Med,* 1982;73:235–238.

Kerby, G.R., et al., "Nocturnal Positive Pressure Ventilation via Nasal Mask," *Am Rev Respir Dis,* 1987;135:738–940.

Law, P.K., B.S. Goodwin, and M.G. Wang, "Normal Myoblast Injections Provide Genetic Treatment for Murine Dystroph," *Muscle Nerve,* 1988;11:525–533.

Lord, J., B. Behrman, N. Varzos, D. Cooper, J.S. Lieberman, and W.M. Fowler, "Scoliosis Associated with Duchenne Muscular Dystrophy," *Arch Phys Med Rehabil,* 1990;71:13–17.

Plough, A., *"Borrowed Time": Artificial Organs and the Politics of Extending Lives* (Philadelphia: Temple Press, 1986).

Rideau, Y., G. Gatin, J. Bach, and G. Gines, "Prolongation of Life in Duchenne's Muscular Dystrophy," *Atica Neurologica,* 1983;5:118–124.

Rideau, Y., L.W. Jankowski, and J. Grellet, "Respiratory Function in the Muscular Dystrophies," *Muscle Nerve,* 1981;4:155–164.

Robins Miller, J., A.P. Colbert, and N.C. Schock, "Ventilator Use in Progressive Neuromuscular Disease: Impact on Patients and Their Families," *Dev Med Child Neurol,* 1988;30:200–207.

Rochester, D.F., N.M.T. Braun, and S. Laine, "Diaphragmatic Energy Expenditure in Chronic Respiratory Failure," *Am J Med,* 1977:163L223–232.

Segall, D., "Noninvasive Nasal Mask-assisted Ventilation in Respiratory Failure of Duchenne Muscular Dystrophy," *Chest,* 1988;93:1298–1300.

Stewart, C.A., I. Gilgoff, A. Baydur, W. Prentice, and D. Applebaum, "Gated Radionuclide Ventriculography in the Evaluation of Cardiac Function in Duchenne's Muscular Dystrophy," *Chest,* 1988;94:1245–48.

Wolff, J.A., et al., *Science,* 1990;247:1465–1468.

2

LIFE WITH DIGNITY—DEATH WITH DIGNITY

Esther Ehrenberg, M.A.

Medical technology has given us choices that heretofore were unavailable. Medical equipment can keep us alive, long after a clinical death is evident. It is inevitable that each individual responds differently to the choices available. Also, various factors have set ideas of protocol, be it physicians, religious groups, or cultural constraints. Recently the question arose as to whether the state may take away an individual's power to control life-and-death issues within its jurisdiction. The Supreme Court is now wrestling with the problem. Just what are the rights of the individual in this controversy?

The United States Constitution provides for "life, liberty, and the pursuit of happiness." Does right to life include an artificially maintained life? Today any individual can ask for and receive all the life-sustaining procedures that the medical profession can offer. As for liberty, does that not include the liberty to decide one's own medical course, or destiny? The pursuit of happiness may well include the quality of life. When deep physical or psychological pain causes one to plead for death, must that one be forced to continue to suffer indefinitely? There is a vast difference between taking a life and allowing nature to take its course; the former could lead to numerous abuses, while the latter may be more humane.

These constitutional rights lead to a dilemma: who decides which rights belong to whom? It is generally accepted that minor children do not have the same rights as adults. The state has laws concerning abuse and child labor, and requires certain inoculations prior to attending school, which is compulsory. The law is now concerned with parents' rights to decide life-and-death issues of their own children. Anyone who has witnessed a terminally ill child suffer agonizing pain would think twice before putting that child on life-sustaining equipment. How then to resolve the issue of parents' rights versus the law?

For adults, the constitution appears to permit freedom to make decisions regarding one's own life. Not so, when the state steps in to allow the courts jurisdiction over an adult's expressed wishes. Unless one has a living will etched onto one's chest, medical personnel must resuscitate and place the patient on life supports or face possible legal action.

Living wills are available from Concern for Dying in New York, and may be registered with this group. Copies should be in the possession of an individual's physician, attorney, and family members. With community support, living wills may become legal in New Jersey.

Today I am presenting a case history of a brave, heroic woman who had amyotrophic lateral sclerosis, known as Lou Gehrig's Disease (ALS). I was called in to assist her in her wish to have her respirator removed and made a home visit to meet with the woman and her family. By that time, the disease had left her with only one means of contact: she could move her eyes from right to left to indicate yes or no. She had gradually, over four years, lost all muscular control, was tube fed and lying in a hospital bed in her living room, surrounded by medical paraphernalia. She required suctioning frequently, day and night, as she could not swallow and could easily choke if unattended. She had no way of calling for help, and was totally dependent upon people asking the right questions for communication. Her husband had arranged for nurses to be present while he was at work. He cared for her during the nights, sleeping on a couch facing her, so he would be on hand if there were any problem with the respirator.

The patient had a clear mind. She was aware of the toll her illness was taking on her husband and children, physically, emotionally, and financially. The entire family lovingly centered their lives around their beloved wife and mother. However, it became difficult for the patient to keep her eyelids open. She knew that when she could no longer raise her eyelids, she would be completely isolated from her husband, her three children, and her grandchild. She would no longer be able to while away the hours watching television, or let anyone know when she needed to be changed, moved, etc. Nor could she ever let anyone know if she were in pain or discomfort. But her mind remained clear.

My first task was to verify the patient's wishes and determine that she was of sound mind and rational. She had contemplated removing the respirator as soon as she could no longer communicate with or see her family. I first saw her in November, and she explained to me she wanted to have one last Christmas and New Years with her family. I spoke separately and privately with her husband and each of her children, and they all concurred with the patient's wishes, feeling that they would have wanted the same for themselves. I suggested that the family and nurses maintain confidentiality until I could research the protocol and questions of legality necessary to help them carry out her wishes. I contacted several organizations, including Concern for Dying, and the medical library, where I read the Hastings Institute report on medical ethics pertinent to my patient's case. In order to protect the patient and the family, we needed to have her attending physician, plus two psychiatrists, attest to the fact that the patient was of sound mind. The attending physician did not make house calls, and the patient was no longer able to be taken to the emergency room of the local hospital for her check-ups. Finding a new attending physician and two psychiatrists who would make house calls was an arduous process taking several weeks to complete. I was present when the new attending physician came, gave the patient a thorough examination, and agreed to accept her as a patient. The physician also spoke with the family members. The two psychiatrists who came also spoke with the family members after they had examined the patient. Each found her to be of clear, sound mind, and testified to that in writing.

At that point, we were able to proceed with the plans the patient had for her death and funeral, both of which were well thought out in advance. She wanted to see her clergyman, which the family arranged, and he agreed to officiate at her funeral. We needed to meet with the entire family at once to finalize the plans. Each part of the planning had to be checked out first with the patient, then with family members for consensus. The only time there was a difference was when the patient indicated she wanted her children to be present at her death. They said they wanted to be with their mother until she was well sedated, but not when the respirator was turned off or she died. That was acceptable to the patient. She also wanted her husband to turn off the respirator, but he was unable to comply. That created a problem, until we found a person who was willing to do it. This delayed the entire plan for a few weeks. A new date was established, so that the patient's mother and other family members from distant parts of the country could arrange travel plans. When all plans were completed, I asked if my services were needed any longer. I was not required by the patient to be present at her death.

Follow-up after one year confirmed that the patient's family had made a good adjustment and was going on quite well.

3

CARDIAC FUNCTION IN DUCHENNE'S MUSCULAR DYSTROPHY

Use of Radionuclide Ventriculography in Initial Evaluation, Progress, and Stress Testing

Charles A. Stewart, M.D.
Irene Gilgoff, M.D.
Guo-Long Hung, M.D.
Rana A. Bahl, M.D.
Ahmet Baydur, M.D.
Radha Sarma, M.D.

Duchenne's muscular dystrophy (DMD) is a progressive muscular dystrophy with severe respiratory and cardiac manifestations. Death is caused by respiratory insufficiency in most cases, but congestive heart failure secondary to cardiomyopathy may be an important cause as well. Advances in assisted mechanical ventilation now offer therapeutic options and some hope of prolonging longevity and meaningful survival for the patient dying of respiratory failure. Thus the detection of myocardial involvement is becoming more important for both the treatment and the prognosis of the patient with DMD. The cardiomyopathy of DMD is well-described (Berenbaum and Horowitz, 1956; Gilroy, et al., 1963; Weisenfeld, et al., 1952). Many studies have reported ECG findings (Perloff, et al., 1967; Slucka, 1968) and echocardiogram findings (Goldberg, et al.,1980, 1982; Hunsaker, et al., 1982) in DMD. While these studies are descriptive of cardiac changes in DMD, they are neither diagnostic nor prognostic. Others have applied radionuclide methods to study myocardial metabolism, perfusion, and wall motion in DMD (Iorio, et al., 1988; Kawai, et al., 1985; Perloff, et al., 1984). Gated radionuclide ventriculography is a reliable means of evaluating cardiac function and determining a left ventricular ejection fraction (LVEF). Since the LVEF is an indicator of global left ventricular function, it should be indicative of the clinical significance of the cardiomyopathy of DMD. We have used gated radionuclide ventriculography in the initial evaluation of DMD cardiomyopathy and have looked at the relationship between LVEF and age, as well as pulmonary function. Gated radionuclide ventriculography may also be used for following the progression of cardiomyopathy, as well as evaluating response to pharmacological or ventilatory interventions. When performed under stress conditions, radionuclide ventriculography may identify patients with insufficient cardiac reserve.

We have previously reported (Stewart, et al., 1988) our initial study of cardiac function as determined by LVEF and its relationship to age and pulmonary function. To date we have performed initial LVEF determinations using gated radionuclide ventriculography in 44 DMD patients ranging in age from 23 years to 42 years (average 23.1), all Swinyard Class 7 or 8. The determinations of LVEF versus age in all patients showed a wide range from 11 percent to 70 percent. By the early twenties, most were found to have LVEF below 50 percent; however, two patients in their early teens had LVEF in the lower forties. Four studies were performed in patients over the age of 30. One had a normal LVEF of 51 percent, two had mild abnormality at 38 percent and 40 percent, and one was 25 percent. While there is a general trend, with younger patients having better LVEFs than older patients, by the mid-teens and early twenties, most patients had LVEF less than 50 percent. Within this group, there was also a wide variation from only mildly abnormal to severely abnormal.

There was no direct correleation between LVEF and age (r=0.197). Some older patients continued to have an adequate LVEF above 50 percent, whereas some younger patients had severe cardiac disease associated with a low LVEF.

All of the patients studied had decreased pulmonary function. Eleven were fully ventilator dependent at the time of initial cardiac evaluation. Twenty-three had pulmonary function evaluation with diminished FVC, average 18.7 percent of predicted range (7 percent to 43 percent). Again a wide range of values for LVEF was seen. Seven patients with FVC of less than 3 percent had a normal LVEF above 50 percent. Two with FVC of less than 13 percent had a normal LVEF above 50 percent. There was no good correlation between LVEF and FVC (r=0.138). In fact, in the fully ventilator-dependent group, for which the FVC could not be determined, the LVEF ranged from 11 percent to 55 percent.

Our study has led us to conclude that no significant correlation exists between the severity of respiratory dysfunction and cardiac function or between age and cardiac function. The cardiomyopathy of DMD, although of the same pathogenesis as the respiratory muscle dysfunction, presents clinically as a separate entity. It is therefore imperative to study each patient's cardiac status when evaluating the options concerning long-term assisted ventilation.

In our initial group, an LVEF of less than 20 percent indicated the inevitable occurrence of irreversible congestive heart failure within one year. Five patients had a LVEF of less than 20 percent, and all died of heart failure within one year of our study of them.

Three were not receiving assisted ventilation and died at three, five, and ten months, respectively, after their first LVEF determination. Two were receiving assisted ventilation for two and five months, respectively. Each died one month after their LVEF determination. From this initial study it could not be determined for how long the LVEF in the five patients had been below 20 percent. In order to determine the rate of progression of the cardiomyopathy of DMD, we have begun to perform yearly LVEF determinations. By closely following the clinical status as it relates to LVEF, we will be able to better determine the true prognostic significance of LVEF changes.

Over 40 patients have been followed for up to four years with yearly LVEF determinations, or more frequently if clinically indicated. Continued follow-up will allow for the determination of the rate of progression of cardiomyopathy. To date, we have identified one patient with LVEF of less than 20 percent who is still alive at 27 months and one who died after 31 months with LVEF less than 20 percent.

Serial studies also allow for documenting changes in LVEF due to therapeutic interventions such as the initiation of assisted ventilation or cardiac pharmacologic therapy. Three patients who required the initiation of assisted ventilation due to respiratory failure. All had mildly abnormal LVEF before ventilation, and all showed an improvement in LVEF after ventilation, probably due to improved oxygenation status. Improved LVEF was maintained for up to two years, but all have now demonstrated a decreasing LVEF back to preventilation levels. Various pharmacologic therapies have been proposed for the treatment of DMD cardiomyopathy. We are currently evaluating several pharmacological protocols. Preliminary data indicates at least an initial improvement in LVEF in five patients treated with low to moderate doses of captopril. Of course, further follow-up is needed, but the usefulness of gated radionuclide ventriculography in assessing the results of interventions is demonstrated.

One patient demonstrated a transient drop in LVEF during an acute episode of pneumonia. This suggests that the patient population may lack a sufficient cardiac reserve to respond to stress. Iorio (1988) studied a younger DMD population by evaluating LVEF and LV wall motion at rest and during handgrip exercise. In most cases a reduction in LVEF with exercise was found. We have recently begun to study the effects of stress on LVEF. Since our patient population is older, with more severe skeletal muscle involvement, and many are ventilator dependent, they are unable to exercise for conventional stress testing.

We have studied three patients at rest and under stress using transesophageal atrial pacing to increase the heart rate and simulate exercise conditions. Two showed a normal response of increasing LVEF with exercise, 47 percent to 78 percent and 36 percent to 54 percent. One patient showed an abnormal decrease in LVEF from 33 percent to 16 percent. We believe this technique may allow for the identification of those patients whose LVEF is adequate under resting conditions but who lack sufficient cardiac reserve to respond to stress.

Cardiac function as determined by radionuclide ventriculography can be used to predict morbidity from DMD cardiomyopathy. No significant correlation exists between the severity of respiratory dysfunction and cardiac function or between age and cardiac function. It is therefore imperative to study each patient's cardiac status when evaluating the options concerning assisted ventilation. Radionuclide ventriculography can be used to follow the progression of DMD cardiomyopathy and to evaluate response to pharmacologic or ventilatory interventions. When performed under stress, radionuclide ventriculography may identify patients with insufficient cardiac reserve to respond to stress.

REFERENCES

Berenbaum, A.A., and W. Horowitz, "Heart Involvement in Progressive Muscular Dystrophy," *American Heart Journal* 1956, 51:622–630.

Gilroy, J., J.L. Callahan, R. Berman, and M. Newman, "Cardiac and Pulmonary Complications in Duchenne's Progressive Muscular Dystrophy," *Circulation* 1963, 27:484–493.

Goldberg, S.J., L. Feldman, C. Reinecke, L.Z. Stern, D.J. Sahn, and H.D. Allen, "Echocardiographic Determination of Contraction and Relaxation Measurements of the Left Ventricular Wall in Normal Subjects and Patients with Muscular Dystrophy," *Circulation* 1980, 62:1061–1069.

Goldberg, S.J., L.Z. Stern, L. Feldman, H.D. Allen, D.J. Sahn, and L.M. Valdes-Cruz, "Serial Two-dimensional Echocardiography in Duchenne Muscular Dystrophy," *Neurology* 1982; 32:1101–1105.

Hunsaker, R.H., P.K. Fulkerson, F.J. Barry, R.P. Lewis, C.V. Leier, and D.V. Unverforth, "Cardiac Function in Duchenne's Muscular Dystrophy: Results of Ten-year Follow-up Study and Non-invasive Tests," *American Journal of Medicine* 1982, 73:235–238.

Iorio, F., M.F. Luzzi, I. Genuini, F. Scopinaro, and A.C. Colella, "Equilibrium Radionuclide Ventriculography in Duchenne's Cardiomyopathy," *Nuclear Medicine Communication* 1988, 19(5): 357–361.

Kawai, N., I. Sotobata, M. Okada, M. Iwase, S. Yamamoto, H. Matsushima, H. Mujakoda, M. Yokota, K. Yamauchi, and H. Hayashi, "Evaluation of Myocardial Involvement in Duchenne's Progressive Muscular Dystrophy with Thallium-201 Myocardial Perfusion Imaging," *Japanese Heart Journal* 1985, 26(5):767–775.

Perloff, J.K., A.C. Deleon, and D. O'Doherty, "The Cardiomyopathy of Progressive Muscular Dystrophy," *Circulation* 1966, 33:625–648.

Perloff, J.K., E. Henze, and H.R. Schelbert, "Alterations in Regional Myocardial Metabolism, Perfusion and Wall Motion in Duchenne Muscular Dystrophy Studied by Radionuclide Imaging," *Circulation* 1984, 69(1):33–42.

Perloff, J.K., W.C. Roberts, A.C. Deleon, and D. O' Doherty, "The Distinctive Electrocardiogram of Duchenne's Progressive Muscular Dystrophy," *American Journal of Medicine* 1967, 42:179–188.

Slucka, C., "The Electrocardiogram in Duchenne Progressive Muscular Dystrophy," *Circulation* 1968, 38:933–941.

Stewart, C.A., I. Gilgoff, A. Baydur, W. Prentice, and D. Applebaum, "Gated Radionuclide Ventriculography in the Evaluation of Cardiac Function in Duchenne's Muscular Dystrophy," *Chest* 1988, 94: 1245–1248.

Weisenfeld, S., and W.J. Messinger, "Cardiac Involvement in Progressive Muscular Dystrophy," *American Heart Journal* 1952, 43:170–187.

4

LIVING AND DYING WITH VENTILATOR-DEPENDENT QUADRIPLEGIA

Frederick M. Maynard, M.D.

Persons with spinal cord injury at upper cervical levels may develop complete quadriplegia and may require continuous mechanical ventilation to sustain life. Until 10 or 15 years ago, few people survived such injuries. With advanced emergency medical services, trauma centers, and broad public training in resuscitation techniques, more people now survive this type of acute injury and require rehabilitation. Several spinal cord injury centers in the United States have developed special programs for the comprehensive rehabilitation of patients with high cervical spinal cord injury with ventilator dependency. There are many unique physical characteristics about this group of long-term ventilator users, such as extensive sensory loss, bowel, bladder, and sexual dysfunction, and circulatory abnormalities. However, the most significant difference affecting psychosocial adaptation between them and chronic ventilator users due to other conditions may be related to the acute onset of their medical condition, which also includes chronic ventilator use.

As a rehabilitationist, I prefer talking about living with spinal cord injury, rather than the problem of dying with spinal cord injury. Nevertheless, both are important and inevitable. Let me begin on the positive side by sharing the statistics on quality of life reported by patients with ventilator-dependent quadriplegia who complete comprehensive rehabilitation at a specialized, model spinal cord injury center program. Whiteneck, et al. (1985) found that 93 percent of patients with high level quadriplegia and ventilator use reported "being glad to be alive." Furthermore, most of them rated the quality of their life as high. It is interesting that quality of life was rated lower by high level quadriplegics who did not use ventilators than by those who did. Most patients in both groups lived at home after completing their comprehensive rehabilitation programs. The programs include all the components of care: physical therapy, occupational therapy, speech therapy, psychology, counseling, extensive family support, and extensive discharge planning. A complete description of state-of-the art methods for comprehensive medical care and rehabilitation of patients with ventilator-dependent quadriplegia has been reported by Whiteneck, et al. (1989).

Suicidal ideation, or the wish to be dead instead of alive after injury, was reported at some time after injury by about half of the patients surveyed by Whiteneck, et al. (1985). The frequency of recent suicidal ideation among this particular sample of patients was only 10 percent. It should be noted that these statistics were obtained from people who completed comprehensive rehabilitation at a specialized center. I am certain that there are many patients who have the same type of physical impairments who die in acute care or who are not referred to specialized centers because of limited insurance sponsorship, social support, or the will to survive. For people who do enter and complete these specialized programs, most will return to community living and achieve a satisfactory quality of life. Necessary medical care, rehabilitation equipment, and maintenance assistance services are expensive and their availability can significantly affect quality of life, especially in regard to personal autonomy. Therefore, availability of and financing for these needs is a major priority for the independent living movement and can be expected to influence a person's attitudes toward living and dying with severe physical disability.

In order to examine the issue of choosing to die after surviving an injury resulting in quadriplegia with ventilator dependency, I would like to describe five cases. All of the people became dissatisfied with their lives and hopeless about their condition. Each made a conscious choice not to continue living, although the circumstances surrounding the decisions illustrate the broad spectrum of factors which may relate to making such a decision. The ethical issues raised by younger individuals with ventilator-dependent quadriplegia who request ventilator removal are sometimes considered unique because their condition is not terminal or progressive. However, current life expectancy after injury for people with complete quadriplegia may be only 33 percent of normal for a person of comparable age (DeVivo, 1990). Although 63 percent of the patients with ventilator-dependent, high quadriplegia reported by Whiteneck, et al. (1985) were alive seven years after injury, most were young and all had survived the first six to nine months after injury and had completed rehabilitation. In regard to the nonprogressive nature of spinal cord injury, Trieschmann (1987) has pointed out that the natural history of long-term quadriplegia is one of progressively more impairments, commonly due to accumulating secondary complications associated with aging. Although spinal cord injury is usually considered a stable impairment, it affects so many of the body systems that a person may be constantly dealing with complications, which in their frequency and totality often lead to progressive disability. Thus, ventilator-dependent quadriplegia may not be so different from other progressive conditions that are commonly considered fatal because of their late stage ventilator muscle involvement, such as amyotrophic lateral sclerosis or muscular dystrophy. The course before death may be more protracted after spinal cord injury, but muscular dystrophy patients now live into their thirties and forties, and the difference between them and a patient with ventilator-dependent quadriplegia whose condition at 20 may be minor. Both can be expected to live until age 40.

CASE REPORTS

Case 1

J.B. was a 17-year-old boy when he sustained a cervical fracture from a shallow water dive in 1982. Initially he showed C5 quadriplegia; the paralysis extended to the C1 level on the third day after injury and he was placed on mechanical ventilation. He spent three months in intensive care units and an additional five months in a comprehensive rehabilitation program. His chronic medical management included not only full-time positive pressure ventilation but a gastrostomy tube, a supra pubic tube, regular turning, a bowel program, and medication for spasticity. He required head and neck support when sitting up and complained of chronic neck pain. Functional rehabilitation included establishing verbal communication with a talking tracheostomy, achieving independent mobility with a sip-and-puff controlled electric wheelchair, and written communication through Morse Code input to a computer using an environmental control unit. All of these activities were successfully incorporated into his home care plan. His parents were very involved with his care. One of them was with him or near his room the entire eight month hospitalization period, even though they both continued full-time employment. They lived near the hospital, and the father had excellent medical insurance benefits. Additionally, friends raised money that allowed an addition to be built on the family home and a van to be purchased and adapted for their son's use. The home discharge plan included 24-hour agency nursing care, although the family also knew how to perform all aspects of his care.

The personal side of the young man's story was that J.B. was a very bright student, a good athlete, and popular with his peers. He had a difficult time becoming involved in his rehabilitation program. About three months after his injury, he had an extensive discussion with his parents about his wish not to go on living. The parents made a "compact" to "give it at least one year to see what life is like in your condition and if after that period of time you still haven't changed your mind, then we are willing to assist you in pursuing some means to end your life with ventilator-dependent quadriplegia." Their discussion was not shared with the rehabilitation team. During the year he was home, he did attend a community college and took a math course. He was able to talk on the telephone, attend rock concerts, and go on community outings. He told jokes and retained a sense of humor. However, he did not change his mind about not wanting to continue living with his condition. He showed little pride in performing the limited functional activities that he was capable of doing independently. He described his life as "perpetual boredom, loneliness, and pain" (Cackley, 1986). He experienced a complete loss of privacy by the presence of nurses around him at all times. He wrote, "this country was founded on the principles that everyone should have the right to life, liberty and the pursuit of happiness. I don't have much of a life nor do I have the means to pursue happiness" (Cackley, 1986).

After the year passed, at age eighteen and one-half, he asked his parents to obtain an attorney who would help establish his right to be removed from the ventilator. A court was petitioned to grant the right to be removed from the ventilator and to immunize caretakers from legal liability or prosecution for homicide if they executed his request. Legal proceedings took about one year. The case was handled privately and was never discussed in the news media (it should be remembered that this action took place in 1984, a different period from 1990 regarding the right to die). J.B. was found to be competent by two court-ordered psychological evaluations. As his managing physician from the rehabilitation center, I agreed with the findings of legal competence and the absence of a depressive disorder. The court petition was eventually granted. Two weeks later plans were made by the family for the home care nurse to leave on a Saturday afternoon. This request was not unusual and did not cause suspicion on the part of the agency nurses that the ventilator would be removed. The family remained alone with their son for a time of remembrance. After saying farewells, his father stayed with him and removed the ventilator. J.B. closed his eyes and died peacefully within three or four minutes. A church funeral was held three days later. The family has coped well since these events. I have stayed in contact with them and they have provided some peer support to another family going through a similar experience. A complete description and discussion of this case has been published (Maynard and Muth, 1987).

Case 2

J.D. was a 30-year-old woman who had a cervical fracture due to a motor vehicle accident and developed high level quadriplegia with ventilator dependency. She was transferred between five acute care hospitals during the first 18 months after her injury. None of these facilities had a comprehensive medical rehabilitation program for people with ventilator-dependent quadriplegia. Since she was an active duty Navy employee when injured, she was transferred to a Veterans Administration Spinal Cord Injury Center that had a rehabilitation program for patients with ventilator-dependent quadriplegia. The family remained distant from the young woman, who was single, and never became actively involved in her care. They never thought it was possible or feasible to have her live with them after the injury. She was a bright woman who had been a computer programmer for the Navy. She became very angry about her condition and care during the acute care hospitalizations and expressed the desire to die. When she entered the rehabilitation program she was still angry and frustrated about having to continue living with her condition. Shortly after admission, she began demanding that the hospital staff remove her from the ventilator. Nevertheless, with a full rehabilitation program that included psychologists, social workers, and therapists, she intermittently did engage in feasible rehabilitation activities. However, on two occasions she removed herself from the ventilator by disconnecting the tubing with neck movements. She argued with the nurses about whether they had the right to force her to continue living by reconnecting the ventilator. This behavior caused extreme distress among the rehabilitation unit staff. Eventually, because of her persistent requests to be allowed to die, mental competency was established by psychiatric evaluation, and the rehabilitation counseling psychologist concurred with the psychiatric opinion. She obtained legal counsel from an attorney affiliated with the institution and the legal office of the Veterans Administration was consulted because of concern about the government's responsibility if a nonterminal patient were removed from a ventilator. After nine months of trying to give this woman hope for the future through rehabilitation, the staff gradually became convinced that not only was she competent, but she had made an unwaivering decision to discontinue living. The staff was not happy with the decision but realized there was no alternative to granting her the right to be disconnected from the ventilator. A conference was arranged, at which the rehabilitation team, as a group, would communicate its decision to grant her request and begin planning for her removal from the ventilator. As the staff began to explain its decision, she snapped off the ventilator. The staff remained calm and several members asked her if she wished to be reconnected. She clearly indicated that she did not. The staff stayed with her until she died. It took a long time for the rehabilitation unit staff to emotionally process this experience, which was shared through a panel presentation to the American Association of Spinal Cord Injury Psychologists and Social Workers (George, et al., 1988).

Case 3

T.S. was a 20-year-old man who was injured while playing soccer in 1975 in California. His impairment was C3 quadriplegia and he required mechanical ventilation. His care took place in a comprehensive spinal cord injury center. He received rehabilitative care over a ten-month period and eventually was discharged into a three-person group home which was created by his mother. She was a nurse and divorced from his father. Following her son's accident, she organized a community fund raising program that allowed her to purchase a house and remodel it as a residence for young men with ventilator-dependent quadriplegia. T.S. was a good student in college who participated in competitive athletics. His family and friends were supportive; nevertheless, he became angry about his physical dependency and began demanding that his ventilator be removed about five months after the injury. One night he secretly enlisted the help of his sister, who disconnected him from the ventilator. They were discovered by the nursing staff and he was put back on the ventilator. This event precipitated a lengthy discussion by the rehabilitation staff and the patient's family. Meetings were held with attorneys, clergy, the rehabilitation team, and the family. No legal action was initiated (it was 1975, and the Karen Quinlan case had not yet come to the public forefront). Eventually T.S. was discharged to the group home run by his mother, although he had remained sullen and passive during his final months of rehabilitation. Two months after he was discharged, he was brought back to the hospital in a coma from a drug overdose. He died two days later without regaining consciousness. It was never ascertained who may have assisted him in taking the overdose.

Case 4

C.D. was a 26-year-old single woman who was injured in a motor vehicle accident in 1989. She sustained a high cervical spine fracture and showed complete C3 quadriplegia requiring mechanical ventilation. She also sustained a skull fracture and was not fully conscious for about three weeks. She spent four months in an acute care setting but was not informed about her prognosis. By the time she was moved from the acute care facility to a rehabilitation center, she had become despondent. She was told at the rehabilitation center that since she had only Medicaid insurance, she would be allowed to remain there only two weeks. The family was given the impression that a change in her attitude was the primary goal for rehabilitation. Although she was supportive, her mother was not able to provide a suitable residence or constant care in a home setting. After three weeks of rehabilitation, the patient was transferred to a nursing home. Prior to her injury, C.D. had worked as a respiratory therapy technician who hoped eventually to enter medical school. Given the circumstance of anticipating permanent residence in a nursing home, she became hopeless. Indeed, she had been given little hope of recovering. The physician at the nursing home who became responsible for the care of this angry young woman was not willing to remove her from the ventilator. He did have a lengthy discussion with her and her family about other options. She had been having recurrent fevers, thought to be pulmonary in origin. The physician did agree to withhold antibiotics during her next episode of sepsis. Within a week, she became septic and died.

Case 5

D.R. was a 20-year-old man who developed C5 quadriplegia in a surfing accident in 1970. During the next 15 years he was able to spend only three periods, ranging from two to six months each, living outside a nursing home. During one period he lived with a female companion who provided his care, but the relationship did not last and he was unable to establish himself in long-term independent living. He did take community college classes while residing in a nursing home. At age 35, he developed post-traumatic cystic myelopathy, a late complication of spinal cord injury that can produce greater neurological impairment. He lost the movement that he had in his upper extremities and the ability to breathe adequately. He was placed on tracheal positive pressure ventilation. There was little discussion with him about the long-term nature of the ventilator use. He spent two months in a spinal cord injury rehabilitation program before being transferred to a nursing home that provided care for ventilator-dependent patients. During rehabilitation, he showed little interest in learning to use available technology for independence. When he returned to the nursing home, he participated in few of the available activities. He rarely got into his electric wheelchair or attended group recreational activities. He largely chose to remain in bed.

After three years of living under these circumstances, he became very dissatisfied. He expressed the wish not to have his life prolonged further with mechanical ventilation and asked to have it removed. His physician, who was also the owner and medical director of several nursing homes, denied his request because he was concerned about negative public opinion which could follow having a patient at one of his facilities removed from life support. The patient described his dilemma to the local news media and obtained legal counsel. I had the opportunity to discuss possible options with his attorney. I advised him that probably the easiest way for D.R. to have his wishes met was to find a place where he could go outside of the nursing home to be removed from the ventilator. When his case was taken to a state court in 1989, it was interesting to observe how rapidly attitudes had changed regarding this issue. The judge stated that he did not need to hear the case in court because no one was questioning D.R.'s competency.

The judge affirmed previous decisions in the jurisdiction that a competent adult has the right to decline continued use of life-sustaining mechanical ventilation. This opinion surprised and pleased both D.R. and his attorney, but it did not resolve the issue of how he was going to die. After numerous discussions, D.R. arranged with an aunt, with whom he had maintained some contact over the years, to provide her home to him as a location for discharge. He also contacted a hospice physician, who had otherwise not known him, to provide terminal care at the aunt's home. He arranged a celebration party with about 20 friends on the day after his discharge from the nursing home. These events were covered by the local news media, including an extensive interview of D.R. by a television reporter who had paraplegia. Volunteer peer counseling was provided by a local community of disabled rights advocates during the last month of his life. Nevertheless, D.R. affirmed his decision and was removed from the ventilator by the hospice physician after receiving sedative medication.

Hopelessness and despondency are emotions that became prominent and persistent in each of these cases. The origins of these feelings were probably unique to each person. In my opinion, they result from attitudes and values as much as circumstance. The unanswerable question that concerned me about the fifth case was "if the thousands of support letters that came to D.R. because of the newspaper articles had included money instead of messages of sympathy, would D.R. have changed his mind relative to discontinuing support?" Similarly, one wonders how much inadequate resources contributed to the decisions to discontinue ventilator use in cases 2 and 4.

Since recent court decisions have made it clear that people who are competent have the right to discontinue ventilator use, physicians must begin to formulate appropriate responses to patient requests for this action. Perhaps they must begin by acknowledging how difficult it is for people working in rehabilitation, who constantly focus on creating optimal quality of life for people with disabilities, to accede to a patient's request to discontinue life support treatment. This is particularly true when they believe a patient could achieve a satisfactory quality of life but seems to choose not to pursue it. Such patients may create strong feelings of rejection in professionals because of the apparent questioning of the value of their activities. Another problem for professionals is their ethical position about the morality of a person taking such action and/or of a professional assisting. At a 1989 Gazette International Networking Institute Conference, A. Ruggeberg (1989), a visually impaired ethicist from Sweden, proposed that there was no person with a physical disability that was so extensive that the person could not end his/her own life without assistance. He suggested that to allow a person with a stable, if severe, physical disability to withdraw life-sustaining treatment reflected an attitude of discrimination and a devaluation of people with disabilities. What is the distinction between permission for this choice and permission for suicidal action by a person who has high level quadriplegia, without ventilator dependency, who becomes despondent with life? When the young man in Case 3 was denied ventilator removal, he did proceed with suicide, which has recently been reported by DeVivo (1990) as perhaps the third most common cause of death among people with spinal cord injuries during the first 18 years after injury. Deciding how to respond to a patient's request to withdraw life-sustaining care is not an easy decision for health care professionals.

I would like to share my ideas about how medical professionals should respond when a mentally alert and competent person with ventilator-dependent quadriplegia requests that the ventilator be removed. Clearly, a quick, simplistic response that "this person is competent in my opinion, so I guess I must honor the request" is an inappropriate response. In my experience, the first thing to consider is whether the patient is expressing suicidal ideation or has made a thoughtful choice to discontinue life-sustaining treatment. I think there is an important distinction between the two notions. As opposed to the 50 percent of patients surveyed by Whiteneck, et al. (1985) who reported suicidal ideas, all of the people in the cases presented earlier had made clear choices that implied, "I want to be taken off the ventilator now and I know what this means." Frequently, requests for ventilator removal are ignored because they are uncomfortable to deal with. Responding to a request to have a ventilator removed in the same way as responding to suicidal ideas may appear to trivialize the request and offend the patient. Sometimes, responding to a request for ventilator removal with a discussion about the common occurrence of death wishes can be helpful and reassure a despondent patient. Misinterpreting a thoughtful request as an expression of temporary depressive thoughts must be avoided.

When it is clear that a patient is serious about requesting removal of a ventilator, it becomes important to acknowledge the legal right of the patient to refuse medical treatment. As mentioned, courts have consistently ruled that competent patients may be removed from ventilators. A battle of wills with the patient should be avoided. I think it only raises a person's resolve to be removed from a ventilator when a doctor says, "we cannot allow you to do this." Such a response accentuates feelings of loss of control, which can be expected to be high among people with extreme physical dependency. When I reflect on the histories of the five intelligent people whose case histories I have described—who came to a common decision to end their lives—it appears they all came to believe they needed to prove that they had the legal right to decide their own fate. This issue became very important to them. J.B.'s parents (Case 1) believe this was probably his primary purpose for living during the last year of his life. During the time his court petition was pending, he had an episode of gastrointestinal bleeding when his hematocrit fell so low he would have died without a blood transfusion. He permitted the necessary treatment at home and was interested in prolonging his life until his court case was won. In my opinion, if a battle of wills can be avoided from the beginning, some people may get through their hopelessness and change their minds about wanting to live. I have had this experience in at least one case. Additionally, the case of McAfee that was reported in *Time* magazine (1990) supports this view, since he has chosen so far not to discontinue ventilator use, even after pursuing permission from the Georgia Supreme Court to do so. Occasionally, distressed patients may try to manipulate staff and family by expressing the wish to die. Taking these patients' requests seriously can sometimes expose a manipulative ploy.

What else should be done, in addition to discussing the right to refuse continued treatment, when a competent patient makes a considered choice to discontinue ventilator use? I think there are several action steps for the patient and several for the professionals. Action steps for patients include the following: 1) obtaining their own independent legal counsel (most patients and families know how to do this and only need permission and encouragement to do so; other patients may need help finding legal counsel, and fees may be problematic); 2) discussing their request with family, significant others, spiritual counselors, etc., having been given ample opportunity to talk with as many people as possible about their current condition and their options for the future; 3) be willing to meet peers and learn about their lives. Who is a peer for these patients? One who has a similar physical condition and ideally is of the same sex, social, economic, and educational background. It may be difficult to find a peer, but anyone who is living successfully while using a ventilator can be helpful, and; 4) learning about the outcome of various rehabilitative possibilities. Specially produced videotapes and other educational sources for patients and families should supplement verbal and written reports of possible goals and of the process needed to reach them. Independent psychological evaluations must be conducted to establish the person's competency to make decisions about his or her condition, the implications of having the request granted, and the options for continuing care.

Action steps for the professionals should include the following: 1) consultation with a medical ethics committee. Most institutions have them, and they provide support for professionals, as well as handle legal questions, since usually attorneys are members of such committees; 2) discussions with all members of the rehabilitation team, so that everyone understands the procedure. Plans should be reviewed so that all team members work together. Everyone's feelings should be acknowledged, and individuals should be reassured that they will not be asked to violate their moral integrity; 3) communication with the patient's family. If there is continued dialogue, opportunity for the patient to change his or her mind about a decision to die can be insured. All interested parties can voice their concerns and severe emotional pain following termination of life support can be minimized; 4) facilitating and enabling the patient to complete his or her action steps; 5) formation of an opinion by the patient's treating physician regarding the patient's capacity to decide about his or her welfare. I concur with the recommendations of the Hastings Center (Smith and Veatch, 1987) that a "process standard" should be used for determining capacity to make such decisions. As rehabilitation professionals we may be appropriately concerned that a patient's decision is a result of temporary reactive depression. We may wonder if a patient is really able to evaluate his or her situation and make a competent decision. Applying a"process standard" can ensure that a decision is responsible and well thought-out. By giving a patient some action steps to carry out, his or her behavior can be observed over time. During this time, when an attorney is being contacted, interviews taking place, information being provided, and a discussion occuring with other people, the patient's capacity to understand the available choices and implications of his or her decision can best be determined by the patient's physician.

In summary, I believe there frequently is therapeutic value in articulating respect for a patient's autonomy and right to refuse treatment as an initial response to a request for ventilator removal by patients with ventilator-dependent quadriplegia. Knowledge that the decision is ultimately theirs may make them likely to change their mind with the passage of time. Patients with strongly expressed desires to withdraw mechanical ventilation may have a high probability of dying one way or another, regardless of what action is taken by professionals. Patients who succeed in having mechanical ventilation withdrawn and reject the life offered by rehabilitation may create strong feelings of futility and low self-worth among professionals. However, the paradigm of independent living emphasizes the central role of individual self-determination, irrespective of physical helplessness. Therefore, when a person who has tested life as a ventilator-dependent quadriplegic after optimal rehabilitation elects to have treatment withdrawn and end life under these circumstances, the decision can be viewed as consistent with traditional goals of medical and rehabilitation practice.

REFERENCES

Cackley, A., "Remember Jimmy Blodgett?" *Ypsilanti Press,* March 16, 1986, p. 1A.

DeVivo, M.J., "Survival After Spinal Cord Injury," *Abstracts Digest.* Paper presented at the annual meeting of the American Spinal Injury Association, Orlando, FL, May 3–5, 1990.

George, J., L. Pearson, S. Mourer, A. Fonseca, and J. Weber, "The Right to Die and Individual Quality of Life Values: The Management of a Patient's Wish to Die," Panel presentation at the annual meeting of the American Association of Spinal Cord Injury Psychologists and Social Workers, Las Vegas, NV, August 29–31,1988.

Maynard, F.M., and A.S. Muth, "The Choice to End Life as a Ventilator-dependent Quadriplegic," *Archives of Physical Medicine and Rehabilitation,* 1987, 68:862–864.

Ruggeberg, A., "Mutual Decision-making in Life and Death Situations." Respondent remarks at panel presentation to Gazette International Networking Institute's Fifth Annual Conference on Independent Living and Post-Polio Rehabilitation, St. Louis, MO, June 1–4, 1989.

Smith, D.H., and R.M. Veatch, *Guidelines on the Termination of Life-sustaining Treatment and the Care of the Dying: A Report by the Hastings Center* (Bloomington, IN: University Press, 1987).

Time, March 19, 1990, "Love and Let Die," pp. 62–71, P. Painton and E. Taylor.

Trieschmann, R., *Aging With a Disability* (New York: Demos, 1987).

Whiteneck, G.G., C. Adler, R.E. Carter, D.P. Lammertse, S. Manley, R. Menter, K.A. Wagner, and C. Wilmot, *The Management of High Quadriplegia* (New York: Demos, 1989).

Whiteneck, G.G., R.E. Carter, S.W. Charlifue, R. Menter, M.A. Wilkerson, and C.B. Wilmot, *A Collaborative Study of High Quadriplegia* (Englewood, CO: Rocky Mountain Regional Spinal Cord Injury System for National Institute for Handicapped Research, Craig Hospital, 1985).

5

IMAGES OF LIFE AND DEATH

Julie G. Madorsky, M.D.
Shirley M. Acosta, M.A.
Daniel Heilburn

This chapter was written by a child who lived and died with Duchenne's muscular dystrophy, his doctor, and his psychotherapist. As such, it is an integration of three different points of view about the psychosocial aspects of this disease.

Daniel was three years old when he was diagnosed as having Duchenne's muscular dystrophy. He was six years old when we made a decision to write a book together. The title of the book was to be *What I Want the Doctors to Know About Muscular Dystrophy*. The book was never written; instead, this chapter collects, records, and analyzes his experiences.

Daniel died when he was 12 years old. He lived the final year with the full knowledge of his impending death. His words and drawings provide a window through which professionals can gain insight into a child's experience of the joys and the sorrows, as well as the challenges, of growing up with muscular dystrophy.

As health professionals, we, the doctor and the psychotherapist, would have liked to shield Daniel from contact with sorrow. We would also have liked to protect ourselves from having to deal with his awareness of his impending death. But instead of giving in to the temptation to participate in a conspiracy of silence, we chose to engage in an ongoing dialogue with Daniel, the results of which follow. We have found similar dialogues about life-and-death issues to be of value with other Duchenne's muscular dystrophy patients, including those who have had an additional diagnosis of mental retardation. It is our hope that this chapter will show clinicians how it is possible to remain supportive and helpful to patients and families through progressive stages of the disease.

No one is an expert in the area of death. The most important thing we have to offer is ourselves: someone who will listen and communicate interest, empathy, and respect, and a willingness to share in the quest for wisdom and understanding.

AGE FOUR

Daniel was first seen by us at age four. He was the product of a normal pregnancy. There was no prior history of muscular dystrophy in the family. He stood at 8 months and walked at 18 months. By the age of four, he was experiencing daily falls that resulted in a broken leg and a concussion.

On examination, he was bright and pleasant. Strength was fair plus proximally in the arms and legs. He had pseudohypertrophy of the calves. There was mild heel cord tightness but no other limitation of motion. He walked on his toes with a slightly broad-based gait and used Gower's maneuver to get up from the floor. CPK was 27,500; muscle biopsy was compatible with primary myopathy.

His father was a salesman, his mother a psychiatric technician. The parents were having marital difficulties that included disagreements on how best to protect Daniel from injury. They were in marital counseling.

Medical recommendations at that time were for outpatient physical therapy to try to reverse heel cord tightness and for resting splints to be used at nighttime.

AGE FIVE

By age five, Daniel walked with bilateral gluteus medius and maximus gait, on his toes with the legs in abduction. He fell several times a day. He used a manual wheelchair for long distances. The parents were in the final stage of divorce.

At this time, Daniel was referred for psychological evaluation and treatment because of stuttering, nightmares, and bed-wetting. During the initial interview, his mother did all the talking; Daniel said nothing. His appearance was quiet and almost wistful. He was disinterested in any of the toys or activities offered. At the end of the interview, he was asked if he would like to come again by himself to play or talk. Surprisingly, he said yes.

Subsequently, he participated in psychotherapy through the media of games, toys, puzzles, songs, and stories. He did not like to talk very much. Drawing pictures became his favorite activity and principal means of interaction.

AGE SIX (See figure 1.)

Daniel drew his first picture [See figure 2.] at the age of six years and four months and then said, "This is what will happen to me." We began discussions that day about muscular dystrophy.

Daniel's first picture was of a person with a face—eyes, nose, mouth, hair, and neck—but without arms or legs. There is a body without clothing, and a mechanical device where there should be feet. The body is encased in some kind of body brace up to the neck. The figure showed no movement.

Intellectual testing at about this time revealed a verbal IQ of 120, performance IQ of 112, and a total scale IQ of 119. Daniel appeared angry and depressed, unable to express his emotions verbally. His drawing appeared to demonstrate a knowledge of his disease and disability and express his sense of hopelessness. Our interpretation was that this child, at the age of six years and four months, had sufficient cognitive development to comprehend what was in store for him.

Arrangements were made to continue play therapy to facilitate exploration of his feelings and verbalization of his grief, despair, and anger. Family therapy with his mother and sister was also planned to try to alleviate some of their stress.

By the age of six years and eight months, muscle strength was in the poor grades proximally and fair grades distally. Ankles were contractured at 20 degrees of plantarflexion; grasp was weak. He walked on his toes with hyperextension of the back, with extreme instability and frequent falls. Surgical consultation was declined by his mother. He was no longer able to propel a manual wheelchair except on smooth, level surfaces. An electric wheelchair was prescribed for him. Respiratory therapy was initiated to build up vital capacity.

By this time, Daniel was no longer quiet or wistful. He talked a lot. He talked about the breakup of his parents' marriage and how much he missed his father. He worried that maybe his muscular dystrophy was the reason his dad had left. He was beginning to wish that he didn't have muscular dystrophy. He started to say that he did not like being handicapped. Stuttering was diminishing. He continued to have problems with bed-wetting and sleep.

[See figure 3.]

This is a picture of Santa Claus. This is me standing on Santa Claus' shoulder. I am asking him if he can make something that will make handicaps go away for me. Santa Claus used his magic to get so big, maybe he can use his magic for me. If there is no magic, then I will just live handicapped. I will be sad, but it will be okay. It is not the doctor's fault; it is God's fault. He is the one who made me handicapped. I don't like it.

Several authors, including Bowlby (1969, 1975, 1980) and Kubler-Ross (1969), have identified discrete stages that a child or adult experiences in dealing with loss. However, Daniel's Santa Claus picture and story illustrate the coexistence of magical thinking, protective denial, angry blaming, acceptance, and acknowledgment. He had some measure of hope that Santa Claus could magically cure him, yet he could accept the probability that if there were no magical cure, he would have to deal with his predicament.

Treatment included acknowledging the appropriateness of his feelings, validating the reality of his experiences, and encouraging the verbalization of his thoughts and the venting of his feelings.

One week after he drew the Santa Claus picture, we saw Daniel again. This time, he was visibly upset.

[See figure 4.]

I have made a picture of my bird. The cat attacked the bird and he died. I was afraid to touch him because he was dead. I think about dying sometimes. I am afraid when things don't move.

Daniel was visibly upset about the bird. He didn't know whether to be mad at the cat or mad at the bird for dying. The picture reflects his confusion about the cat and the bird. It was only while Daniel was dictating the story that it became clear that the real problem was his awareness of his own potential death. By this time, he had determined that it was all right for him to talk about these things; the therapist could handle it.

Although the psychiatric literature indicates that until age 10 children can accept the idea that someone else has died but cannot understand that they, themselves, might die, it is clear that this child, at the age of six years and seven months, not only acknowledged the reality of death in general but had an understanding and fear of his ultimate demise.

AGE SEVEN

When he was seven, Daniel's mother became aware of information published in the medical literature that some improvement in muscle strength had been noted in a few patients with Duchenne muscular dystrophy who were given Allopurinol. She requested that Daniel receive trial doses of the medication. She was informed about potential side effects of the drug, and a trial was agreed to. At this time, Daniel's strength was in the poor to fair plus grades. He had no evidence of scoliosis, but a molded body jacket for prevention of scoliosis was recommended. A prescription for a hydraulic lift for transportation of his electric wheelchair in the family van was provided.

By the age of seven years and three months, Daniel had acquired his mother's mood of hopefulness regarding the trial of Allopurinol. Yet he also verbalized his awareness of his physical deterioration and that he was afraid. His stuttering was intermittent; sleep problems were lessening; he continued wetting his bed.

[See figure 5.]

Saturday I won two gold medals at the Special Olympics. I am not mad at God or the doctors anymore. I am scared that my handicap is getting worse. I'm not that strong anymore. I'm scared about what's going to happen. I think I can stop my handicap if I try hard enough. I can do it. I can make a formula. All you take is a few things like vegetables and soak them in hot water and it might work. Something will work if I try hard enough. I'm not going to give up.

His picture and the accompanying story express his mood of hopefulness and his emerging sense of a burgeoning internal locus of control. Now, instead of looking to powerful outside forces, such as Santa Claus or the doctor, to cure him, he was exploring his own resources for helping himself. He was beginning to get a sense of his own competence and power. He wondered whether his success in the Special Olympics might be indicative of his potential to overcome other obstacles, such as his disability.

He was encouraged to express his thoughts and feelings through storytelling and drawings and to use his emerging problem-solving skills to gain a sense of control over his handicap.

Just one month later, at the age of seven years and four months, when Daniel arrived he was very angry. He had fallen while playing and could not get up, and no one heard his cries for help. He had lain outside for a long time. He didn't like that. He did not like what was happening to him. He was no longer sad about it; he was mad!

[See figure 6.]

This is a picture of a spaceship blowing up the hospital. I am mad at the hospital because they haven't stopped my handicap. It's been since I was one year old, so it's been seven years. I wish they could stop it. I am mad at the doctors. I want them to stop it. It's making me less strong all the time. I don't know what it will be like in seven more years. I am scared about that.

Clearly, Daniel was in touch with feelings of frustration, anger, and fear about his progressive decline and the lack of a cure. He was encouraged to express his anger and to explore the realistic options for using his remaining capabilities to live as full and active a life as possible.

AGE EIGHT

At age eight, Daniel was doing well in school academically. Mainstreaming him from an orthopedically handicapped school to a regular elementary school was being explored. Muscle strength was in the poor minus to poor plus grades. He could feed himself, write, and draw; however, he needed assistance for all other activities. Fifty degree hip flexion contractures and 20 degree knee flexion contractures were present. He could no longer wear shoes due to the discomfort and pressure created from his equinovarus foot deformities. He was getting visibly weaker physically, but was happier emotionally. He was happy about the freedom afforded him by the electric wheelchair. His father began to spend more time with him. School was going well. He went to City Hall to complain that the push buttons on the traffic signals were too high for wheelchairs. They listened, and he felt good.

[See figure 7.]

I am lucky because I get to do neat things like going for a ride on the blimp. I did that with my dad for my birthday. I can't do things that other kids can do, but sometimes I can do things that other kids can't do. I can't run or climb or walk. I can still use my hands. I would like to do all of the things that I can't do. I hope they find a cure for muscular dystrophy pretty soon.

By this time, Daniel had stopped bed-wetting and stuttering and was sleeping through the night without bad dreams. Our assessment was that he was no longer depressed and that he was adjusting appropriately to his disease and progressive disability. At the same time, he was able to acknowledge the potential to enjoy life and find happiness in his ability to participate in various activities with his family and peers.

It was agreed that plans should proceed to mainstream him into a regular elementary school. Further, it was recommended that regular psychotherapy sessions stop and be scheduled on an as-needed basis only. Meanwhile, he would continue to have regular medical checkups.

AGE NINE

By the age of nine years and three months, Daniel was attending an orthopedically handicapped class in a regular elementary school. He was an A student. He was assertive with his sister and classmates in fighting for his rights and needs.

Strength was in the trace to poor grades. There were 60 degree hip and knee flexion contractures. The ankles were fixed in severe equinovarus deformities. There was a slight thorcolumbar scoliosis present. Vital capacity was 33 percent of norm. He was gaining weight. He developed small pressure sores. A mechanical lift was used for transfers between bed and chair. He used mobile arm supports to exercise his upper extremities. He was no longer able to draw.

> *I went to the dentist's office yesterday. It was fun. They checked my teeth and cleaned them. I had no cavities. Brushing my teeth has gotten harder and harder. I can't raise my arms anymore. I can move my feet and toes. I can move my head. I can move my mouth a whole lot, and I do. I can move my eyes. I can wiggle my nose. Except for my arms and legs, the rest of me works pretty good. My mouth works best and most. My mind works too. It thinks a lot. It thinks about so many things, I can't even tell you. Sometimes it thinks about things that make me frightened. Dying is the most frightening. If I didn't have muscular dystrophy, I think I would live until I was eighty. I hope I will live until I am eighty anyway. I am afraid that I will have to die.*

Despite Daniel's progressive physical limitations, he was blossoming in his capacity to value his assets, including his skill in engaging in meaningful interpersonal relationships. Concurrently, his willingness to face up to the inevitability of death was increasing. Discussions were begun about the option of ventilator support later, if needed. Additionally, we validated for him that his acceptance of death did not mean giving up; it meant recognizing death as the culmination of life. We planned to remain available to him whenever he chose to reach out for support, comfort, and closeness. We encouraged him to continue to enjoy life. Additional adaptive equipment, such as a hospital bed, was prescribed to facilitate the tasks of daily living.

AGE TEN

By the age of ten, Daniel's head control was poor. He knew he was growing weaker. School became increasingly important to him, as he discovered that there he could shine. He was proud of his academic achievements and excited when the school recommended that he skip sixth grade and start junior high school.

> *My birthday was on March 21, 1984. I turned ten years old. I started writing these stories when I was six. I was having trouble then coping with muscular dystrophy. I was scared. I knew that in a year or so I wouldn't be able to do a lot of things. I felt different from the other kids. I wanted friends, but everybody thought I was different. I didn't know how to tell them that I wasn't different. I also used to feel mad, but I didn't know who to be mad at. Sometimes I thought about being mad at God. If it hadn't been for Him, I wouldn't have been born. Sometimes I was mad at the doctors because that's how I found out that I had muscular dystrophy. There was a time when I was mad at myself because I couldn't keep my feet on the ground and I was always*

on my knees from falling. Sometimes I felt sad. Sometimes I had bad dreams. Something would always come after me and I couldn't get away.

Now most of the time I am happy that I still have what I have. It could be worse. Being stuck in the hospital in one of those iron lung machines would be worse. If it happens, I will be mad and scared and sad all over again. I have about ten years until it will happen. Most people like me live until twenty or twenty-one. That's not long enough. If I could change something, I'd change the time and live longer. It's worth it to be alive and to be here.

At the age of ten, Daniel appeared to be reviewing his life and stages of adjustment. He was able to acknowledge his impending death while putting his energies into living with enthusiasm and gusto. He was considering the potential advantages and disadvantages of ventilator support.

A headrest was prescribed for his wheelchair. We offered to remain accessible to him as he continued to struggle with life-and-death issues.

AGE ELEVEN

At eleven, Daniel underwent bilateral heel cord lengthening procedures. He wanted the operation because he wanted to be able to wear shoes when he transferred into junior high school. Unfortunately, the surgery did not go well, and he was left with chronic pain in the ankles. He was angry and sad following the surgery.

AGE TWELVE

By the age of twelve years and three months, Daniel was so weak that there were days when he could not hold his head up. He needed help turning pages. He had to be fed, dressed, toileted, and bathed. He could not stand the feeling of helplessness and was angry at the boys who teased him at school by switching off the power on his electric wheelchair, thus tampering with his sense of security and control. His academic performance continued to be excellent; however, he was labeled "emotionally and socially immature" by school officials because of expressions of frustration with his peers.

[See figure 8.]

People don't know how hard it really is to be in a wheelchair. You can't walk up stairs and curbs. You can't reach very far. You can't get a drink of water yourself when you want one. You can't go to the bathroom by yourself. It's frustrating! It's embarrassing to ask for help. Sometimes I get mad at myself because I can't do it for myself. I have to hide how mad I am. I have to do that a lot.

Other kids don't understand what it is like to be in a wheelchair. They fuss with my chair. That makes me mad at them. The wheelchair is like part of me. It's how I move from place to place. When they touch the chair, it feels like they are touching me. Sometimes it makes me scared. I am scared of getting hurt or of crashing the wheelchair. If somebody messes with the control and somebody else gets hurt, I get blamed.

At this time Daniel began to withdraw from his peers, as well as from his medical caregivers. He had decided against the option of life support. He was facing death.

The junior high school he attended recommended that he skip eighth grade and go directly to high school. We supported the recommendation, as well as the decision made by Daniel and his mother that there be no heroic medical intervention.

At the age of twelve years and nine months, Daniel turned in his English assignment for the semester, a fifteen-page story about an old man who had been murdered. Daniel's comment at the end of the story was, "It doesn't matter how you died, Ole Joe. The only thing that does matter is how you have lived."

Daniel died in his sleep the night he completed the story. His mother called us right after she called the paramedics. The following morning, she and the family came in to talk, and we planned a memorial service together. At his mother's request, we called the high school to request permission to hold the memorial service there. There was a graveside service also. Daniel's therapists, teachers, and family all told favorite stories about Daniel. His wheelchair was there; the other orthopedically handicapped students had decorated it with balloons. At the conclusion of the service, each one present took a balloon and released it into the air. We said good-bye and let Daniel go.

Daniel's mother and sister continued to participate in family therapy to help deal with Daniel's death and continuing their lives.

CONCLUSIONS

Health care professionals often have mixed feelings about discussing progressive disability and death with children who have Duchenne muscular dystrophy. Often it is assumed that these youngsters are not old enough to understand the issues cognitively and that they are not mature enough to deal with them emotionally. Yet discussions over time can clarify realities and provide opportunities for sharing experiences and feelings by patient, family, and professionals. As mentioned above, it is helpful for health care professionals to acknowledge that no one is an expert on death. It is normal for them to feel anxious and helpless in the face of the imminent death of one of their patients, especially a youngster.

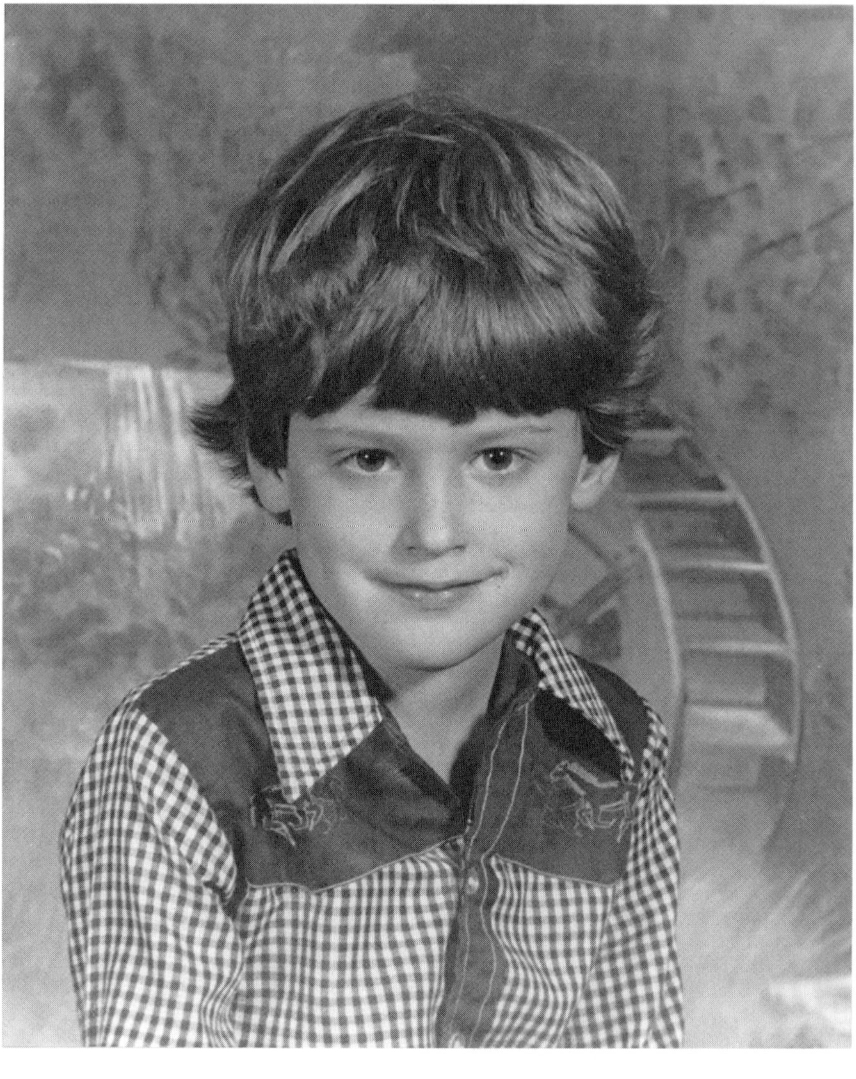

Figure 1. Daniel, age 6

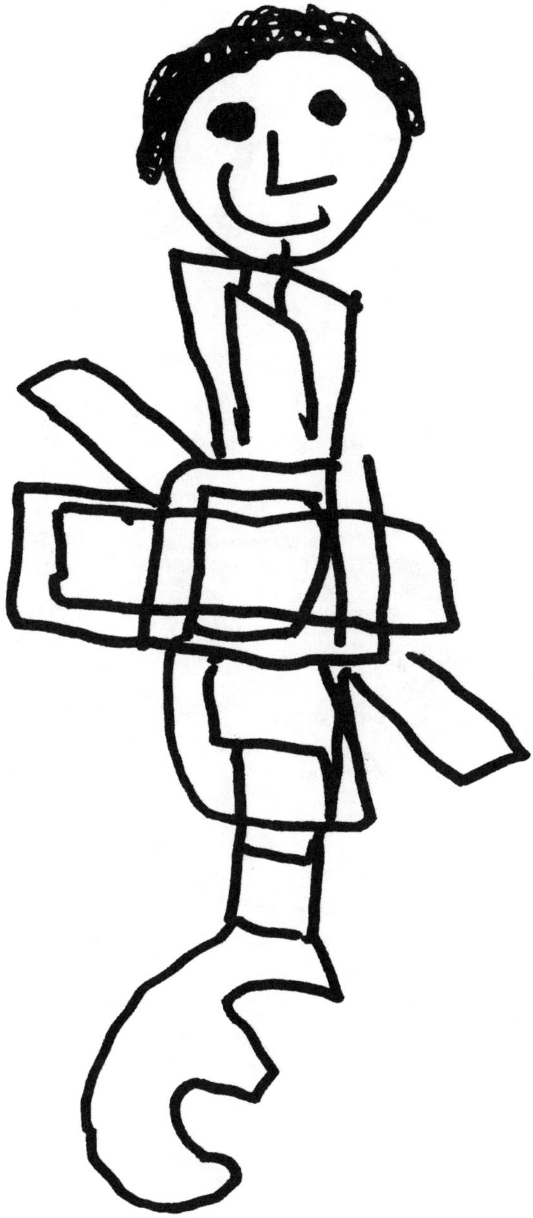

Figure 2.

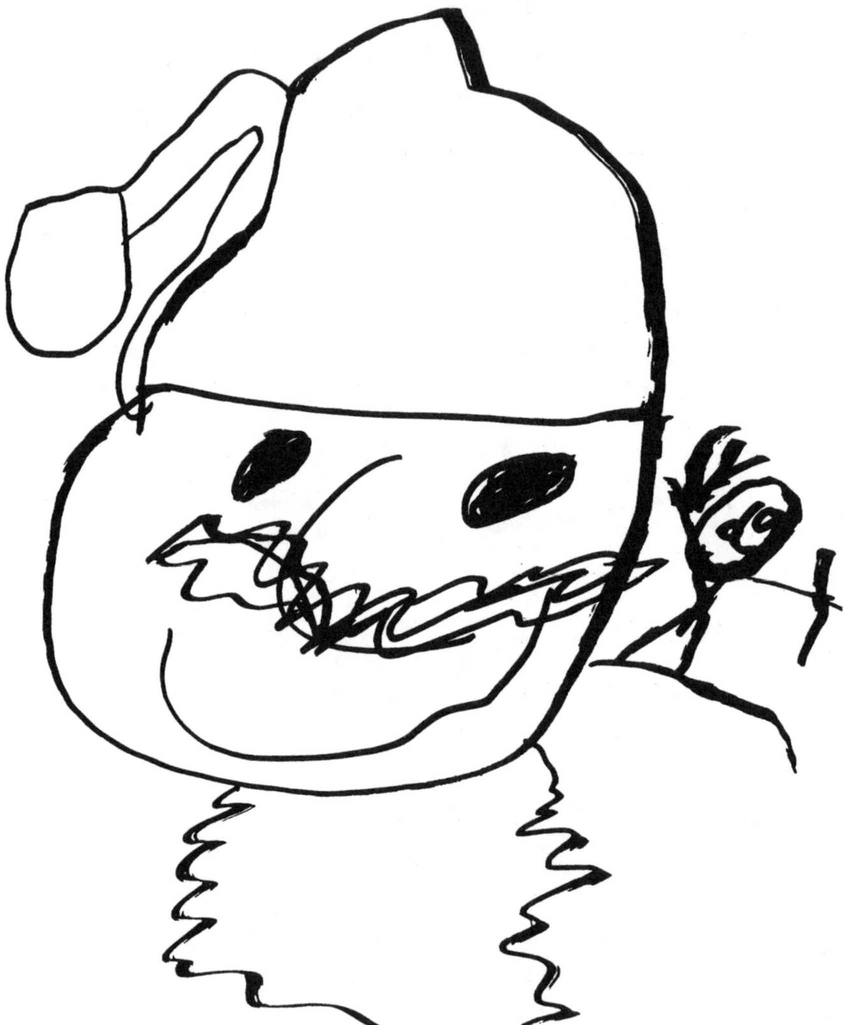

Figure 3.

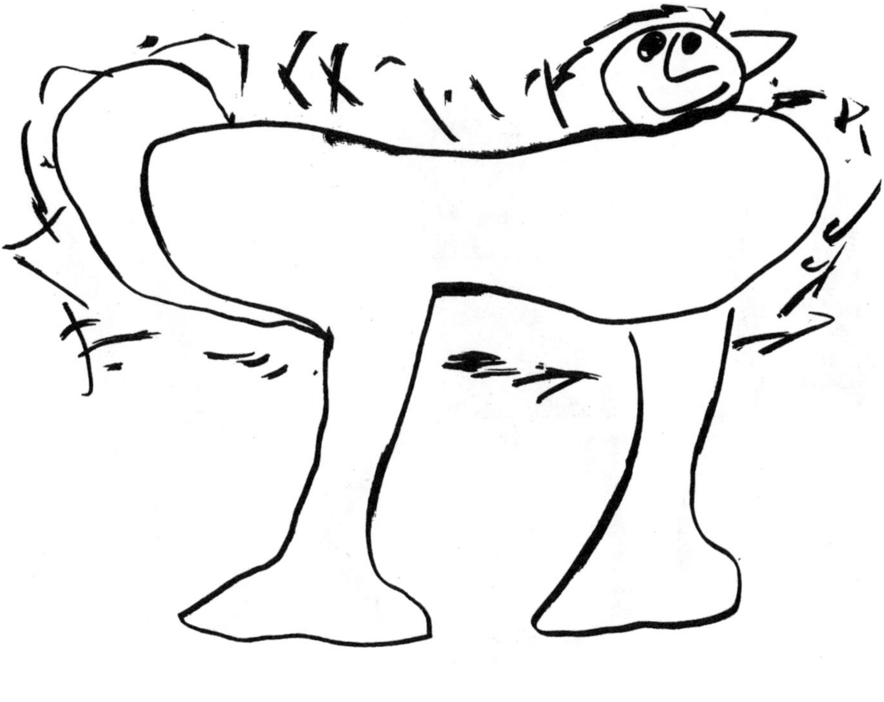

Figure 4.

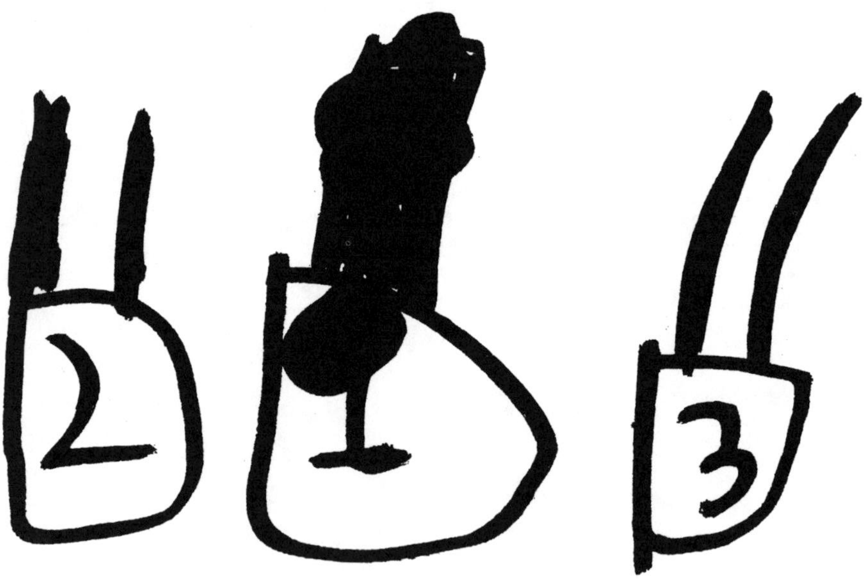

Figure 5.

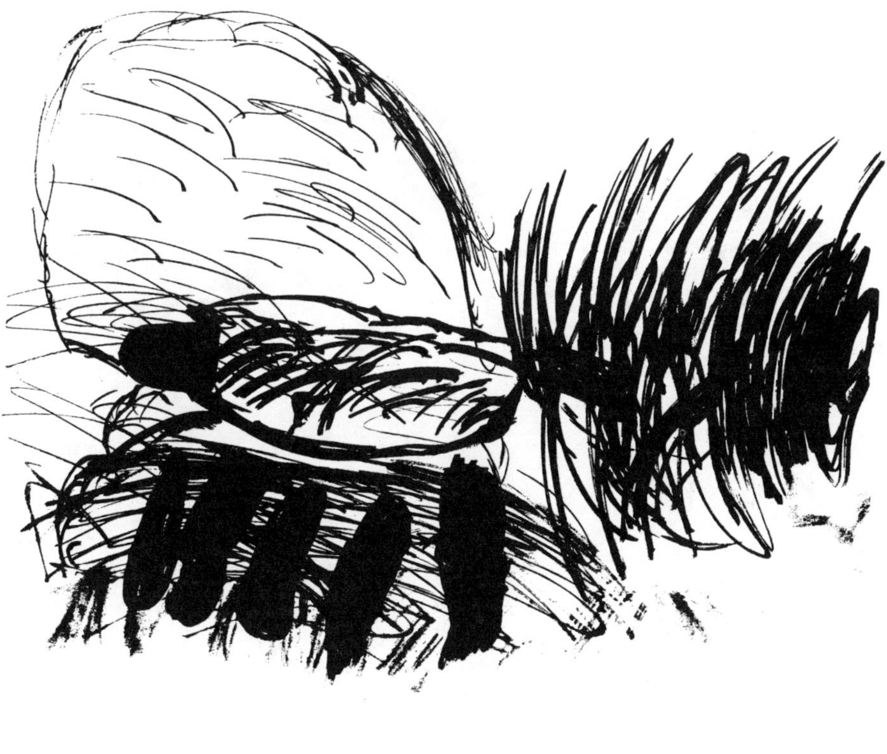

Figure 6.

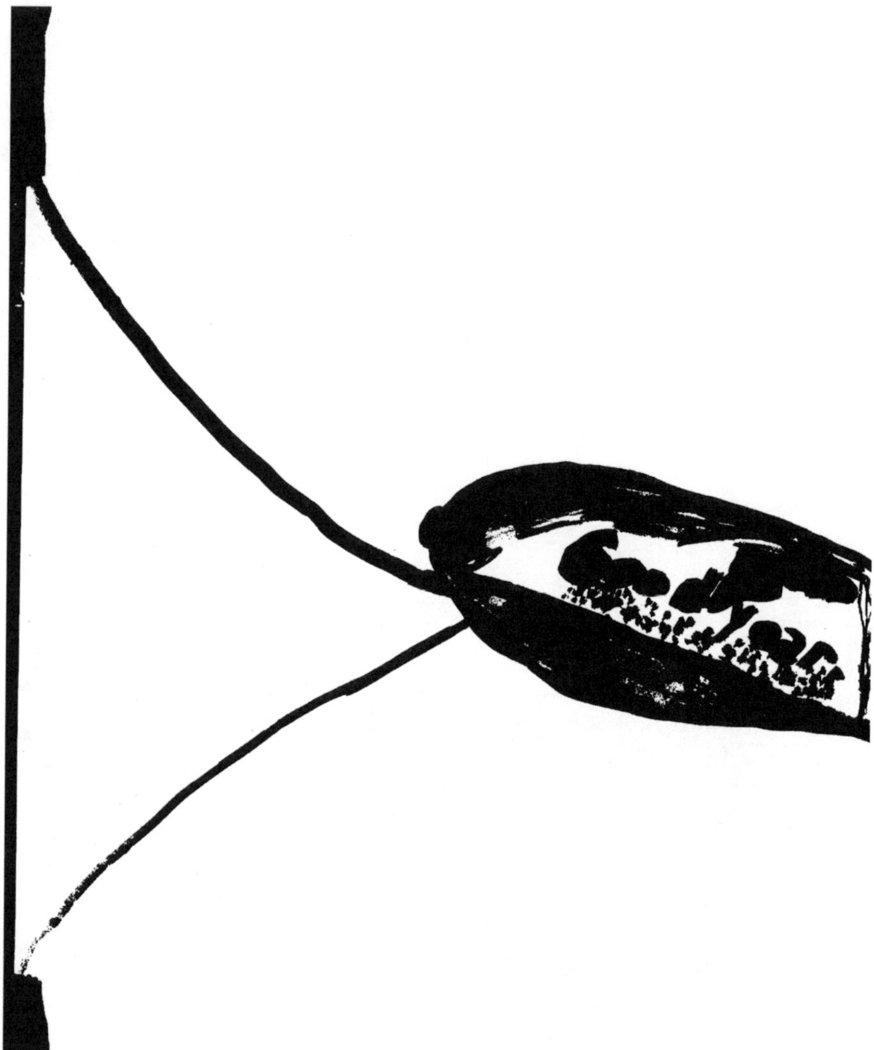

Figure 7.

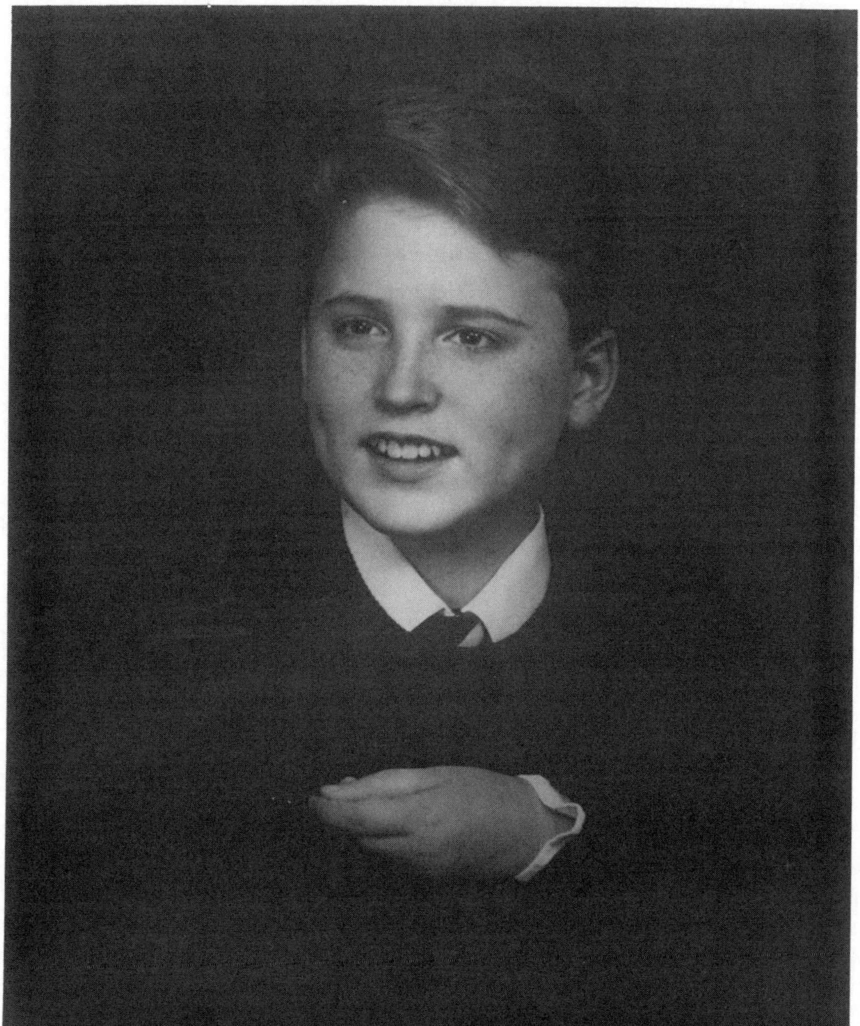

Figure 8. Daniel, age 12

Since, as health care professionals, we are trained to enhance life and fight death, we may experience the death of a patient as a personal failure and an unacceptable conclusion to the health care process. Interestingly, the most frequently observed physician reactions to the death of a patient are anger, denial, and depression, the three most common reactions of patients to their own impending death.

Although a team of health care professionals may be helpful, the physician is the key member of the staff and *must* remain involved. The physician must not withdraw when he or she no longer feels useful. The physician must assure the child and the family that he or she will not desert them. The physician must be honest with the patient and the family, taking the time to explain the tests and procedures to be performed, communicating with siblings, nurses, and other team members the necessary components of supportive care.

In the literature on the subject, there are a number of models that seek to simplify the stages of grieving. Our experience highlights the need for an individualized approach and care plan.

During the development of programs for the psychosocial care of the Duchenne's muscular dystrophy patient, it is essential that each patient's and family's individual needs, preferences, and desires be respected. Interventions should be discussed with the patient, the family, and the treatment team. The religious preferences of the patient and his or her family must be respected.

In planning treatment to meet the needs expressed by patients and their families, it is recommended that an effort be made to maintain the patient as the subject of concern and not as an object of program dynamics. There should not be an attack on denial of death in the name of openness, nor should the patient's right to accurate information be negated. By being emotionally accessible to the patient and the family over time, the physician and the team of professionals can be available when the patient and family choose to acknowledge the possibility of death and the fear of dying.

It is at this time that the option of ventilator support can be gently discussed and assessed. Some patients and their families may view ventilator support as a welcome escape from the probability of death, an avenue of hope for an ongoing creative and meaningful life despite physical disability. Others may perceive it as a means of prolonging an intolerable condition, a living death from which reprieve can rarely be achieved without lengthy battles with the medical and legal establishments.

Decisions regarding possible mechanical ventilation are best made before respiratory failure occurs—by the patient, family, and their trusted advisors—not in an emergency room, with strangers. Daniel's story illustrates the process by which he and his family came to understand his progressive neuromuscular disease and the available treatment choices, and how, in a supportive and caring environment, they responsibly exercised their ultimate right to self-determination.

REFERENCES

Bowlby, J., "Childhood Mourning and Its Implications for Psychiatry," in S. J. Harrison and J. F. McDermott, *Childhood Psychopathology* (New York: International University Press, 1975).

_____, Vol. I: *Attachment* (New York: Basic Books, 1969).

_____, Vol. III: *Loss* (New York: Basic Books, 1980).

Kubler-Ross, E., *On Death and Dying* (New York: Macmillan, 1969).

Madorsky, J.G.B., "Breaking the Conspiracy of Silence Toward Death in Duchenne Muscular Dystrophy," in Leon I. Charash, et al., *Psychosocial Aspects of Muscular Dystrophy and Allied Diseases* (Springfield: Charles C. Thomas Publishers, 1983).

6

THE VENTILATOR

Psychosocial and Medical Aspects

Karen Dikeman
Marta Kazandjian

The role of the speech-language pathologist in the treatment of the ventilator-dependent patient necessitates a broad understanding of communication impairments, as well as medical and pyschosocial issues. This chapter will attempt to provide the reader with an understanding of the impact of communication deficits on the nonspeaking, ventilator-dependent patient. By the very nature of ventilator dependency, patients become communicatively impaired. As communication specialists, we focus on providing the patient with an opportunity to express his or her intentions and concerns, even when the patient is completely nonspeaking.

The importance of the speech pathologist's role in the overall communicative management of the ventilator-dependent patient is best illustrated by a discussion of our involvement on the Bioethical Committee. In our facility, the Bioethical Committee was developed to address patient right-to-die issues. The Bioethical Team at Goldwater consists of the Director of Rehabilitation (an MD), the attending psychiatrist, a psychologist, patient advocate, lawyer, clergyman, social worker, and speech pathologist. As a member of the team, the speech pathologist evaluates the nonspeaking patient who is unable to make his needs known verbally and determines the patient's communicative competency. Communicative competence requires that the patient demonstrate consistent and reliable responses to questions posed by the examiner. The goal of determining communicative competency and mental competency is to assess the patient's capacity to make decisions regarding his or her medical care, including right-to-die (determination) issues. As an example, a patient in the Intensive Care Unit (ICU), ventilator-dependent and aphonic, may require only the provision of an alternative communication system (such as a letter/alphabet board) to indicate his or her wishes concerning medical care. Communicative competency is easily established in such a case. However, a patient with physical, cognitive, and linguistic deficits may be limited to a yes/no communication system. Even in this case, the speech pathologist often can assist in determining the reliability of the patient's communication. At this point, the psychiatrist on the team can proceed with an assessment of the patient's competency and capacity to make decisions. Often the speech-language pathologist (SLP) remains throughout the evaluation, to assist in modifying the language used to a level that a linguistically impaired patient can understand.

There follows a review of the types of communication impairments which might prevent a patient from communicating with the Bioethical Team. The ventilator dependent patient may present with voice, speech and/or language deficits. These deficits, referred to as aphonia, anarthria, and aphasia, span the continuum of disability. Aphonia is the inability to produce voice, possibly due to intubation or tracheostomy and ventilator dependence. Articulatory skills, oral motor abilities, and language skills are usually normal in the aphonic patient. Anarthria, a motor speech disorder, refers to the absence of speech due to severe muscular weakness of the speech mechanism. Language skills are usually normal in the anarthric patient. In contrast, aphasia is a language impairment. All aspects of language, including expression, comprehension, reading, and writing may be impaired to varying degrees in the aphasic patient.

Now look at where a patient's communication deficits fall on the continuum of disability. When assessing the communicatively impaired, ventilator dependent patient, the speech-language pathologist must evaluate the patient's speech/voice, physical motor, and cognitive-linguistic abilities. Consider the speech continuum. At the beginning of the continuum a patient has normal voice production. Vocal intensity and oral motor ability are within normal limits. As you proceed across the continuum, vocal intensity decreases and the coordination of phonation with ventilation is poor; ultimately the patient presents with aphonia. Speech or oral musculature remains intact. Past this point, impairments in oral motor strength begin to emerge. This is where the various levels of dysarthria are demonstrated. Dysarthria is an impairment of speech resulting from muscular weakness. At the end of the continuum, the severest form of speech and voice impairment is illustrated by aphonia and anarthria. We have also made reference to the patient's swallowing deficits, referred to as dysphagia, on the continuum.

Another aspect of impairment that must be considered in the SLP's assessment is nonspeech physical motor status. At the beginning of the continuum, the patient demonstrates good upper extremity range of motion and endurance. As you proceed, upper extremity function weakens and limitations in range of motion are apparent. Eventually, quadriplegia or pentaplegia is demonstrated. It is important that the speech-language pathologist be aware of physical motor status because motor function will later dictate the type of communication system the patient is able to use. For example, a nonspeaking patient with good upper extremity function may be able to write, while a pentaplegic and anarthric patient may be limited to an eye-gaze system for an alternative means of communication.

Finally, assessing cognitive-linguistic status is integral in determining the patient's functional communicative ability. A patient may present with various levels of impairment, from status within functional limits to profound deficits.

These three aspects of impairment, speech, physical motor, and cognitive, make up what is called the continuum of disability. Patients may fall at various points of each continuum. Where they fall on the continuum designates their level of disability. To illustrate how a patient falls on the continuum, we will provide some examples. First, a patient with a diagnosis of COPD. This is a patient who has suddenly become aphonic secondary to recent tracheostomy and ventilator dependence. Articulatory movements are within normal limits, therefore, the patient would be aphonic with good mouthing. Physical motor status may place the patient somewhere between good and poor endurance with good upper extremity range of motion and good fine motor movement. The patient is not expected to demonstrate cognitive-linguistic impairment, since neurological damage did not take place. In another example, the patient status post MVA, who has sustained a high spinal cord injury, may be ventilator-dependent, aphonic, with a mild-moderate dysarthria, and quadriplegic. Dependent upon the presence of head trauma, this patient may exhibit some degree of cognitive impairment. In contrast, the ALS patient illustrates the progression down the continuum as he or she starts out with speech and physical motor status within functional limits but over time deteriorates and is no longer able to move hands, legs, and speech musculature. The patient is aphonic, anarthric, and respirator dependent, yet is cognitively intact.

Our intervention with ventilator-dependent patients is based upon their level of disability, as assessed on the continuum. Intervention methods may be oral, emphasizing the restoration of voice and speech, or nonoral, utilizing alternative/augmentative communication methods. In one type of oral intervention, voice may be restored to the aphonic patient, whose speech and cognition are intact, by means of an artificial larynx. The artificial larynx acts as a source of voice. As an example, a ventilator-dependent patient who also has paralyzed vocal cords may be a candidate for an artificial larynx. Modifications of the tracheostomy tube, such as use of a special "talking tracheostomy," can also restore voice production abilities.

A talking tracheostomy is used with the ventilator-dependent patient who has a cuff that cannot be deflated. An external source of air circumvents the ventilator and provides air to help the patient speak. Patients with both aphonia and dysarthria may need long-term intervention, using oromotor exercises combined with other methods of intervention, to improve speech production abilities. However, for the aphonic and anarthric patient, restoration of speech may not be an option. Such a patient is provided with an alternative/augmentative communication system, a nonoral intervention approach. Augmentative systems can be adapted to address the range of impairments on the continuum of disability. A patient with upper extremity function can write or use a direct selection electronic device with a keyboard. A mini-typewriter is one example of a device which allows a patient access to the keyboard simply by pressing the appropriate letter. A quadriplegic patient may be limited to the use of a mouthstick or single switch when using an electronic device. Severely impaired patients may utilize an eye-gaze system. Any consistent motor movement may be used to link a patient to an augmentative device.

Management of the ventilator-dependent patient can best be illustrated by some case examples. We will refer to the continuum of disability as we discuss communicative impairment and bioethical concerns.

CASE 1

Eugene was a 61-year-old man diagnosed with AIDS and (L) CVA. The patient's communication disability was aphasia and severe dysarthria. He had been receiving speech and language treatment; however, due to a severe depression, he had been refusing all therapy. Prior to his reinitiation to a treatment program, his medical status had deteriorated significantly. His physician and the patient advocate called us for an urgent consultation in order to assess the patient's communicative competency. The psychiatrist and family were also notified. The physician required consent from the patient to proceed with intubation and establish a patent airway. Recall the continuum of disability. Upon evaluation we found the patient's inability to speak secondary to his severe dysarthria.

In terms of physical motor status, he had upper extremity weakness with gross movement of one arm. He was known to present with at least a moderate nonfluent aphasia. Restoring the patient's speech was not an option, due to his aphasia and poor medical status and the urgency of the physician's request. A simple augmentative system was therefore used. We looked for a reliable motor movement the patient could use to indicate yes or no. We had him point to the word *yes* or the word *no* printed in large letters on a clipboard. In establishing communicative competence, we progressed from simple, concrete questions such as, "Are you a man? woman? Are you sick? Well? Are you in a hospital? Movie theater? Are you having trouble breathing? Do you know that the doctor can help you breathe?" to more abstract ones, such as, "Do you know that if the doctor doesn't help you, you will die?" It should be emphasized that during this evaluation the doctor first briefed us on the nature of the information needed from the patient. The psychiatrist was also present and participated in the evaluation. However, the questions were phrased for the comprehension level of an aphasic. Our role was to establish communicative competency for a reliable yes/no response. The physician was then able to determine competency and obtain consent for intubation.

It should be understood that during this crisis intervention, there was no time to think or talk about other options. We had to determine quickly what this patient was capable of deciding. The patient ultimately decided to accept intubation. The family member present was extremely distressed by the decision. It was hard for us to witness the patient's and family member's distress. However, to the best of our ability, we had established communicative competency and provided the means for the patient to communicate his wishes to the psychiatrist and the physician.

CASE 2

Terry was a 27-year-old man diagnosed with ALS, respiratory insufficiency, and quadriplegia. Upon admission, Terry presented with severe dysarthria and received G feedings. Terry had been living at home and was studying architecture. He was also an avid photographer who would select his subjects and then would direct other people in the mechanical aspects of taking the pictures. He made the decision to enter our long-term respiratory unit as the progression of the ALS made it impossible for him to remain at home. He had already explored vocational options. With the help of a speech language pathologist, Terry had acquired an IBMXT computer, which could be accessed through methods other than the keyboard. The computer would allow Terry to continue his vocational goals as he used specific software designed for architects. His speech ability had deteriorated so that oral methods of intervention could not be explored. Our main goal was to train Terry in methods of input designed for his computer. In his case, he accessed the computer via Morse Code. He was also trained in the use of an eye-gaze system, the Eyelink, to communicate with the nursing staff and his family. Terry also used the computer as a writing tool. He wrote poems and letters, many of which described his experience as a nonspeaking person. His motivation to continue with his life probably was best illustrated by the amount of energy he put into insuring that his photography be shown before he died. About eight months before Terry's death, he had an exhibit at a gallery in Manhattan, which illustrated his work as an artist. The speech-language pathologist provided him with an electronic system to use while the many interested observers asked him questions.

Terry had numerous concerns that were relevant to the Bioethical Committee. He had established a do-not-resuscitate order and executed a living will. He not only did not want a tracheostomy and mechanical ventilation, but essentially refused all life-prolonging procedures. As his disease progressed, he was no longer able to access his computer. His eye-gaze system became his only link with the staff and his family. Eventually, at the end stages of the disease, Terry made requests to change portions of his living will. Again, the speech language pathologist was called in to insure that Terry's messages were correctly interpreted. Since Terry had been a patient for two years, the staff had close emotional ties to him. The impact of his deteriorating communicative ability on the staff was great. Even we, as trained speech-language pathologists, had difficulty communicating with him. Terry died according to his wishes, without any of the life-prolonging methods he had declined.

CASE 3

Stephen was a 35-year-old man with a diagnosis of ALS, respiratory insufficiency, and quadriplegia. His case illustrates long-term rehabilitation of a patient with a degenerative disease. Upon admission, Stephen was aphonic secondary to 24-hour ventilator dependence. He was eating a regular diet and was cognitively intact.

Initial intervention was straightforward. Modifications of the tracheostomy tube and ventilator allowed the patient to achieve voice. Oral motor abilities were within normal limits. The patient was also provided with a letterboard which he accessed through a mouthstick, since his head movement was the only motor movement available. He used the letterboard usually at night, when voice could not be achieved. Within two months Stephen's condition got progressively worse, and he became anarthric, aphonic, and dysphagic. Restoration of speech was not an option due to the severity and progressive nature of the disease. When he became too weak to use the mouthstick and letterboard, an eye-gaze communication system (Eyelink) was used. He was also taught to use an electronic communication device for writing.

Stephen used the electronic communication device to print messages to staff and family. Daily, the messages were saved for his wife, children, and brother. Since communication was a slow process and staff found it hard to interact with him, he often expressed frustration with his limitations. At one point he spelled out, "The worse thing about this [his disease] is that I can't even ask for the simplest thing. Every word is agony." The emotion that was poured into these messages by this severely disabled young man, expressing his extreme frustration, was very moving.

As the patient's condition deteriorated, his dysphagia worsened. However, Stephen initially refused alternate feedings. Therefore we consulted with the Bioethical Committee regarding Stephen's case. Because he was nonspeaking and relied solely on augmentative methods of communication, we served as his translator for the doctors and patient advocate. The Bioethical Team met periodically to discuss Stephen's case. Stephen had already established a DNR and had executed a living will. As his physical status deteriorated, the living will was revised as the need for other medical procedures arose.

Stephen was one of our more emotionally draining cases. However, we were able to provide this aphonic, ventilator-dependent, and cognitively intact young man with a way to communicate through the end stages of ALS. The ability to communicate provided some quality of life, as independence was reflected in the ability to make choices.

To conclude, we would like to stress the role that the speech pathologist has on a rehabilitation team dealing with a ventilator-dependent patient. When communication is affected, and it often is, our role is vital. In essence, without communication, the patient is completely isolated. The speech language pathologist's role is to provide the link between the nonspeaking, ventilator dependent individual and his or her communicative partners. We hope that we have increased awareness of the role that the speech-language pathologist plays in the management of the ventilator dependent and communicatively impaired patient. We hope that the speech-language pathologist will be added to the list of those professionals who may be interested in sharing ideas and experiences about these complex patients.

7

THE IMPACT OF VENTILATION TECHNOLOGY

Contrasting Consumer and Professional Perspectives

Joseph Kaufert, Ph.D.
David Locker, Ph.D.

This chapter contrasts the perceptions of technology among polio-impaired ventilator users and rehabilitation professionals. Life historical interviews were recorded with ten people with post-polio respiratory impairment to document the impact of their experience with changing ventilator technology. Ten professionals (respiratologists, respiratory therapists, and respiratory equipment specialists) involved in the care of ventilator users were interviewed to document their perceptions of client adaptation to changing technology. Ventilator users' accounts emphasized adaptive strategies through which the benefits of each successive generation of technology were maximized and social costs minimized. Professional descriptions of clients' history of ventilator use were more fractionated and concentrated primarily on the periods of acute care and changes in vital capacity.

THE LEGACY OF GINI LAURIE IN FOSTERING INFORMATION SHARING BETWEEN PROFESSIONALS AND CONSUMERS

Our interest in understanding the differences between consumer and professional perspectives on ventilators owes much to the vision and inspiration of the late Gini Laurie and the members of her international network (GINI). The GINI conferences and *Rehabilitation Gazette* yearly issues fostered significant exchange of information about alternative methods of risk management and technical data about new generations of ventilation technology. At a 1988 meeting on community based respiratory home care in Toronto, Gini described the exchange which had gone on between consumers and providers in pages of the *Gazette and International Ventilator Users Newsletter.* She emphasized the importance of fostering an open exchange in which the professional made accessible clinical and technological information and the consumer contributed his or her personal experience. Gini Laurie noted that, although current literature documented consumer perspectives, it had not documented the changing perspectives of respiratory rehabilitation professionals. She stressed that professionals could provide a historical sense of the development of technology and evolution of community-based respiratory care. Mrs. Laurie identified the need for an oral history of the pioneering network of health professionals and consumers who were involved in developing the original respiratory centers and home-care programs across North America. This more global project has yet to be developed. However, in the Manitoba follow-up studies of post-polio respiratory impairment, we adopted Gini's concept of asking rehabilitation professionals to describe their experience with succeeding generations of respiratory support technology. We were able to identify the network of respirologists, intensive care specialists, rehabilitation engineers, respiratory therapists, and technologists who were involved in providing respiratory support for the client group between 1952 and 1990. These professional informants were interviewed to document the perspectives of those who provided technical support and care over four decades characterized by rapidly evolving technology.

CONSUMER AND PROFESSIONAL PERSPECTIVES ON VENTILATION TECHNOLOGY

Several others have emphasized that ventilator-dependent survivors of the polio epidemics of the 1940s and 1950s are the first generation of consumers who have lived from childhood to late middle adulthood depending on mechanical ventilation for survival. By exploring the psychosocial, technical, and logistical approaches polio-impaired people used to live independently, a body of qualitative data was generated which may be applied to the experience of ventilator users with other forms of impairment.

This chapter will focus upon the interface between the individual consumer, the professional, and the sociocultural context in which machine and body meet. Conventional views regarding the social meaning of medical technology have emphasized two dominant themes. Professional and public perspectives on life-support technology frequently portray it as an expression of the power of science and mastery by medicine of the process of life and death. More critical approaches from the social science and consumer literature emphasize the hazards of medicalization and loss of control. Part of this literature characterizes medical technology as a negative force, transforming the nature of medical work and influencing both the consumer's and provider's experience of medical care. Unfortunately, neither of these polar perspectives adequately describes the experience of respiratory-impaired people who rely on life-support equipment.

We will briefly summarize respirator users' and professionals' descriptions of the impact of ventilation technology upon life adaptations. In other publications we have emphasized the tension between enabling and handicapping elements of technology (Locker and Kaufert, 1988). We have also considered consumer strategies for balancing advantages and disadvantages of successive generations of ventilators (Locker and Kaufert, 1988). Data from in-depth interviews with professionals and ventilator users will be used to demonstrate how differences in the acceptance of new technology have been influenced by changes in knowledge base and values.

Speakers at a GINI conference on the late effects of poliomyelitis emphasized that some professionals have a selective awareness of the full scope of respirator dependent persons' adaptation during all phases of their use of ventilators. Less knowledgeable professionals were described by consumers as lacking a sense of continuity and awareness of the full range of options for treatment and independent living in community settings. These limitations may reflect the fact that physicians, respiratory therapists, and technologists were selectively involved in the polio-impaired person's care over discrete phases in their adaptation.

METHODS

Data were collected during a follow-up study of survivors of the major Manitoba poliomyelitis epidemics of the 1950s (Alcock, et al., 1984; Kaufert and Kaufert, 1984; Kaufert, et al., 1985). The project included an audit of medical records from the time of the epidemics and two surveys.

Out of the 186 individuals who had been placed in tank respirators, 29 people continued to require mechanical ventilation for more than 12 hours per day. Ten people were selected from this group and interviewed in depth. Five were women and five were men. All had major limb disability in addition to respiratory impairment. The majority had been in their mid- to late twenties at the onset of polio. At the time of the interviews, their ages ranged from 39 to 66.

The people interviewed were selected on the basis of their familiarity with a variety of methods of mechanical respiratory support and their shared experience with rehabilitation medicine and respirology. Five had spent extended periods as inpatients in a large public hospital, and five had lived most of the past 20 years in the community, using services from a home care program.

We are currently in the preliminary stages of collecting and analyzing interview data on professional perspectives on ventilation technology and its influence upon achievable quality of life. To relate the perspectives of clinicians to the life experience of the original sample of ventilator users, we interviewed ten physicians, respiratory therapists, and respiratory technologists who were involved in providing care for the ten respirator users.

In collecting life historical data from people with post-polio residual disability, our initial concern was neither with the impact of technology nor with differences in consumers' and providers' criteria for evaluating functions and quality of life. However, these issues became our main focus when pilot interviews revealed significant differences between users' and providers' perspectives on the quality and character of their everyday lives. Changing technology shaped consumers' biographies in that most discrete changes in their adaptation and perceived quality of life were described in relationship to the advantages and disadvantages of each new generation of technology. Both consumers and professionals described how changes in their perceptions of "optimal use" of ventilators were influenced by their personal and professional values and priorities. For example, user values about maintaining control over maintenance led many to value reliable, user-friendly approaches to ventilation such as the rocking bed or chest shell ventilation. Young respirologists frequently characterized these forms of ventilators in terms of their lower levels of efficacy and lack of technological sophistication.

QUALITY OF LIFE AND DISABILITY CAREERS

Although the concept of a "disability" career provides a useful conceptual framework for considering changes in consumers' adaptation, methodological and conceptual problems are encountered in comparing professionals' descriptions of adaptation with the consumers' total description of their life experiences. Most professional involvement with post-polio ventilation problems was limited to restricted phases of the patient's medical history. For example, respirologists initially involved during the polio epidemics in supporting people in iron lungs frequently had minimal experience with contemporary positive pressure ventilators. Intensive care physicians and respirologists involved in caring for people with late-onset post-polio-related respiratory insufficiency were often less familiar with and accepting of negative pressure ventilators. The perspectives of professionals who were selectively involved in providing care during sequential stages of technology development were expressed in terms of their preference for specific types of ventilators and particular models of care provision (such as hospital-based respiratory care centers or consumer directed respiratory home care). There were also differences between professionals who had experience before the implementation of Canada's comprehensive national health insurance in the 1950s and those involved in providing services under the universal national health insurance system.

In examining consumer and professional descriptions of living with the support of a ventilator, we will examine how life priorities were transformed over the life course as a result of the interplay between personal and contextual factors.

THE "ACUTE" PHASE

Professional and consumer descriptions of the impact of life-support technology upon the quality of life during initial acute care emphasized themes of courage, forbearance, and individual sacrifice among both patients and care givers. Pivotal events in patient interviews centered on the death of patients in adjoining respirators and references to members of the attending clinical staff who were stricken with polio. During the initial period of from 3 to 18 months, in which the respondents were confined to an iron lung, the dominant priority was survival. The dominant psychosocial theme in descriptions of this stage was uncertainty about the degree of recovery achievable and prospects for return to community living. Several ventilator users described uncertainty about the prospects for recovery of functional capacity for mobility and self-care. They indicated that this post-acute experience had been crucial in dealing with personal and clinical uncertainty that had shaped their more current response to the uncertain prognoses of late effects.

Two respirologists who had been involved in providing initial life support and respiratory rehabilitation during the 1952 and 1953 polio epidemics emphasized the logistical problems of providing minimal ventilator support for over 200 patients. They emphasized the reliability and effectiveness of the iron lung in acute care situations. Among the sample of younger intensive care physicians and respiratory therapists who had become involved in ventilatory care after 1970, the post-polio patient's acute care experience in an iron lung was described primarily in terms of baseline measures of initial impairment and vital capacity. The initial experience in an iron lung was perceived primarily as an element of the psychosocial portion of his or her medical history. Perception of efficiency and user friendliness also varied with the generation of the clinician. For example, several of the younger respiratory therapists and intensive care physicians commented that they could not understand why patients continued to resist the adoption of more technologically sophisticated and physiologically efficient ventilators and rejected ventilation through the use of an uncuffed tracheostomy.

Professional norms defining acceptable levels of risk and effectiveness for delivery of ventilator care in the community contrasted with the perspectives of consumers. Respirologists and one of the three respiratory therapists stressed the need to maintain standards for technological support and clinical standards for asepsis in the home care setting comparable to those maintained in intensive care units. In contrast, ventilator users and some older professionals emphasized that their long-term experience with first and second generation ventilators in home-care settings had conditioned them to accept higher levels of risk and uncertainty that maximized patient control and allowed the user to self-direct his or her care within the community.

Following recovery from the acute phase, the respondents entered a period of rehabilitation during which they and professional providers worked toward the recovery of vital capacity and independence in self-care and mobility functions. Interviews with both ventilator users and professionals emphasized the significance of initial acceptance of the rehabilitation model in terms of both quality of life and long-term adaptation. For both patients and providers, the rehabilitation model provided a significant set of values that governed the relationship between the individual and technology and gave meaning and symbolic significance to both.

In their life histories, many ventilator users emphasized that acceptance of the rehabilitation model and decisions about alternative types of ventilators and home care options were largely controlled by professionals. Several ventilator users indicated that they felt the rehabilitation experience had imposed a single model of recovery and long-term life support. This model of successful recovery was perceived by ventilator-dependent patients as not recognizing individual preferences or differences in functional capacity and economic or psychosocial resources. Two respirologists and one respiratory therapist involved in post-acute rehabilitation described the survival and adaptation of a number of ventilator-dependent patients in terms of commitment to the rehabilitation ethic. They emphasized the importance of being a "fighter or survivor" as the principal predictor of successful long-term adaptation among ventilator-dependent patients. Respirologists and respiratory therapists also acknowledged that some elements of the rehabilitation ideology emphasizing avoiding dependence upon supportive technology became dysfunctional in terms of individual adaptations to late aging effects.

For both professionals and ventilator users, the rehabilitation model emphasized maximizing functional capacity, minimizing the use of various forms of support technology, and the importance of individual effort and perseverance in achieving personal and clinical goals (DeJong, 1979). The model also emphasized values such as independence and achievement, which aided both short- and long-term adjustment to mechanical ventilation. However, emphasis upon competition and total independence from support technology in rehabilitation also maximized the possibility of frustration, self-blame, and a sense of moral failure among individuals who did not achieve a high level of functional recovery.

In our life historical interviews, most ventilator users recalled their initial commitment to the rehabilitation ethic and described how they set goals for themselves and persevered until they were realized. Weaning and transition to other forms of ventilators took place in the setting of rehabilitation hospitals that encouraged competition as a therapeutic tool. Emphasis on comparison and competition was perceived by both patients and professionals as having positive and negative sides— false expectations as to what an individual might achieve or depression among those who gauged their performance against the less severely impaired. One woman described being frustrated with her lack of progress: "I thought it must be something I'm doing wrong and other people are doing right."

During the rehabilitation phase, the major index of quality of life, for both patients and professionals, was defined in terms of attainment of respiratory and functional independence. Dependence upon mechanical ventilation technology was sometimes perceived as an impediment to such independence, and as indicative of moral failure.

POST-REHABILITATION PHASE

During the post-rehabilitation period, the level of many of the ventilator users' respiratory function remained relatively constant, although respiratory infections often necessitated a return to mechanical support and hospital care. Stable adaptations in the post-rehabilitation period often were not emphasized in the professionals' accounts because, after the closure of major respiratory centers, many former patients lived independently, with minimal contact with clinicians. For both providers and patients, the primary formula for maintaining quality of life was the admonition to "use it or lose it." This value was later called into question as people began to experience late effects.

TRANSITIONAL PHASE

The period of stability lasted approximately 10 to 15 years, after which most subjects entered a transitional phase characterized by an unexpected decline in respiratory capacity attributed to the late effects of poliomyelitis. Declines in respiratory function associated with late polio-related aging effects brought into sharper contrast the assumptions of the initial rehabilitation model and the physiological and social imperatives of daily living. For patients, this resulted in a change in attitudes, adoption of more effective and portable ventilators, and a fundamental reordering of life priorities.

Both patients and professionals indicated that the acceptance of each new generation of ventilators, with associated benefits and costs, depended on both parties rethinking some of the primary tenets of the early rehabilitation model. The adversarial position implied in patient and professional metaphors referring to "fighting disability" and avoiding dependence upon machinery or other people had to be modified. Emphasis on independence from life-support technology was replaced by emphasis on the quality of life and recognition of the appropriate role of ventilators in achieving this goal. Younger intensive care specialists and respiratory therapists who worked with ventilator users recently have indicated that they were initially puzzled by the reluctance of the polio-impaired patients to accept newer ventilators. Several such professionals indicated they had subsequently learned to listen to their patients' experience with older technology before prescribing new technology.

DEPENDENCE PHASE

Among the ventilator users we interviewed, all had transferred to positive pressure ventilators since 1983, using uncuffed tracheostomies, mouth sip tubes and, more recently, masks for night ventilation. With the exception of one individual, all indicated that the benefits of the new equipment outweighed its cost.

In interviewing health professionals, marked generational contrasts were found between physicians and respiratory therapists who favored tracheostomies and those who favored other methods of connection. Some physicians with ICU backgrounds were willing to provide positive pressure ventilation only through a trachestomy because it was perceived as more efficient. Another physician explained that he had gradually come to accept alternate approaches to connecting a patient to the machine with a mask or mouth tube. He attributed his change in perspective to encountering patients who had successfully used these methods.

THE PERSON AND THE MACHINE

The final transition to modern portable positive pressure ventilation brought with it a different set of problems and constraints. Some of the costs and benefits are attributable to the new body/machine interface, while others are indirect, the result of a changed relationship to the physical and social environment and to the self. Those who used portable positive pressure equipment talked of a new sense of bodily well-being. Both professionals and patients emphasized that the individual's physical and psychological health improved substantially and, combined with increased mobility, transformed the quality of everyday life.

There were discrepancies between patient and professional perspectives on control of technology and training for equipment failure. The users emphasized that the new generation of portable respirators included improved safety features, such as back-up systems and self-monitoring circuits controlled by microcomputers. However, many of these new technological innovations brought new problems. It was reported that microprocessors malfunctioned in below zero weather. In response to the uncertainty of technology, individuals learned to recognize problems before the crisis stage was reached. Patients were sometimes taught little about these problems or the methods of managing them. Rather, problems emerged in the course of daily experience and solutions were found by trail and error. As a consequence, the machine, and tending to the needs of the machine, became the central focus and activity of everyday life. Moreover, the problematic aspects of living with the machine did not detract from its role of promoting a quality of life of more than minimal tolerability.

The accounts of both professionals and patients of recent transitions to modern portable ventilators also emphasized many common themes. The difference in the perception of the quality of life was so dramatic that portable ventilator users often tried to persuade other post-polios to make the transition too. A transformed sense of self accompanied the new dependence upon machinery and the changed relationship to the environment and the people in it. This resort to total respiratory dependence coincided with the final rejection of the rehabilitation ethic that had been the guiding principle of the respondents' lives during the early years of disability.

CONCLUSION

This chapter has used data from a small number of cases to explore the shifting relationships between changing systems of ventilation technology, changing patient needs, and changing culturally based ideologies. A specific set of technologies designed to manage a specific inventory of functional limitations and assess their impact on individual adaptation and quality of everyday life was examined. Although the in-depth life historical analysis of ten individuals has been linked with the more systematic epidemiological follow-up of the total respirator-dependent population in Manitoba, our respondents had a limited spectrum of functional impairments and were cared for in a single system of rehabilitation and long-term respiratory care. Given these limitations, the conclusions drawn are not necessarily generalizable to other groups and service delivery systems. The Manitoba pilot study needs to be followed up through the comparative analysis of other samples of respirator-dependent people. Parallel studies need to be conducted among other cohorts of polio-impaired respirator users and people with other forms of respiratory disability living in a wide variety of care settings.

Despite these qualifications, our preliminary study raises fundamental questions about the contradictory assumptions about dependence upon technology in rehabilitation ideologies, which often are modified as people develop pragmatic adaptations to their changing needs. Among our respondents, the contradictory themes in rehabilitation ideology of avoidance of dependence on aids and adaptation and acceptance of the liberating effects of life support equipment were gradually reconciled as they adapted to the changing ventilation needs of middle age. For both the patient and the professional, improved mechanical ventilation technology was appropriately seen as an effective way of restoring or enhancing respiratory capacity, improving energy levels, and ensuring survival in the short and long term. However, the integration of technology and a chronic disabling condition involves balancing the freedoms and constraints imposed by life-support systems. While the benefits conveyed by positive pressure ventilators were substantial, they were only realized at a cost. Improvements in energy, mobility, and well-being were weighed against the imposition of new routines, new management strategies, and new worries and concerns. In most cases, these benefits and costs were balanced to produce significant and dramatic changes in the pattern of everyday life. The nature and extent of the gains and losses experienced by the respondents appeared to be influenced by variation in individual functional status and the degree to which people were able to modify culturally grounded beliefs about dependence upon technology.

Finally, we have attempted to convey something of the complexity of illness careers by looking at the conflict between rehabilitation ideology and attitudes toward technology, the way this conflict was played out across stages of one chronic condition, and the way it structured immediate life priorities and the broader experience of illness.

REFERENCES

Alcock, A., J. Hildes, P. Kaufert, and J. Kaufert, "Respiratory Poliomyelitis: A Follow-up Study," *Can. Med. Ass. J.* 130, May 15, 1984: 1305–1310.

DeJong, G., "Defining and Implementing the Independent Living Concept," *Independently Living for Physically Disabled People*, ed. N. Crewe and I. Zola (1983), pp. 4–27.

Kaufert, J., J. Syrotuik, et al., "Epidemiological Issues in Follow-up Studies of the Impact of Poliomyelitis," in *Late Effects of Poliomyelitis*, ed. L.

Halstead and D. Wiechers (Miami: Symposia Foundation, 1985), pp. 135–152.

Kaufert, P., and J. Kaufert, "Methodological and Conceptual Issues in Measuring the Long Term Impact of Disability: The Experience of Poliomyelitis Patients in Manitoba," *Soc. Sci. Med.* 19(6), 1984: 609–618.

Locker, D., and J. Kaufert, "The Breath of Life: Medical Technology and the Careers of People with Post-respiratory Poliomyelitis," *Sociology of Health and Illness* 10(1), 1988: 24–40.

8

AUTONOMY, PERCEPTION, AND EMPOWERMENT

Issues in Achieving Quality of Life for Ventilator-Dependent Individuals

Audrey J. King, M.A.

One of the dilemmas in understanding and interpreting issues relating to ventilator dependency is that there are two different cultures, that of the ventilator user and that of bio-medical personnel who provide services and support. These two groups often come with quite different perceptions of what the issues, problems, and solutions are. To gain a true and comprehensive understanding of what ventilator dependency means, it is critical that both the consumer and the professional be heard and that neither presume to speak for the other. Unfortunately, this seldom happens and service providers continue to speak for ventilator users and their families, repeatedly presenting only a "patient-oriented" focus with all its depressing details. Important knowledge about the full, rich, minimally medicalized life that some individuals achieve is consequently missed and positive knowledge, invaluable for the newly ventilated patient, is lost.

There is an assumption by society at large and therefore by those who have not experienced otherwise, that ventilator dependency is a living death, that it means high-tech, high-cost, skilled and dedicated ICU care of patients who are mere bodies—helpless, ill, dependent, and suffering.

This single-scenario drama is perpetuated by the media. These stories sell. This is the knowledge and experience base of most health care providers, for training typically occurs in critical care settings, where life or death is the issue and knowledge of successful ventilator life in the community is absent. Unfortunately, it is this view which also drives policy and the ethical decisions which impact on those using or about to use a ventilator. Not only is this wrong. It is damaging to ventilator users, health care providers, and the community.

There is a need to balance the more common knowledge of "worst" scenarios with a knowledge of how and why some individuals live a full life in spite of severe disability. No one can accurately pre-assess the experience. Geoffrey Spencer, medical consultant responsible for ventilator services in the UK, once asked ventilator-dependent post-polio patients about the quality of their lives. Almost without exception, they said, "If I had known this was going to happen, I would have begged you to take no heroic measures. But now, thirty years later, life has never been so meaningful nor so precious."

Those providing ventilator support need to know and understand this. Physiology and diseases of lungs are taught in medical school. "Living" with dependent lungs is not. Only those who live successfully with long-term ventilator dependence can teach us this.

My acquaintance with achieving ventilator users around the world, my own personal experieince, and my many years of experience as a pediatric rehabilitation psychologist, have led me to conclude there are factors which seem to determine a quality of life so very positive that the greatest fear is denial of the "right to live" in situations of medical emergency.

One of these factors is developmental. If ventilator dependency occurs during youth there is a greater likelihood of achieving adaptability and resilience. Self-perception and social roles are still evolving and malleable. The psychic energy of youth enables one to see things differently and accept new ways of coping. Life's purpose lies still ahead. Goals of relationships, education, vocation, and "full participation within society" drive a younger person towards adaption and adjustment. This assumes, of course, an underlying stability of basic general health.

The longer an individual lives successfully with a ventilator, the less a preoccupation it becomes and the more its relative importance is measured against ordinary aspects of living and goal setting. Acquired skill and experience in managing physical needs and equipment enable this to occur. Given such developmental truth, it is ironic that children with neurological diseases are often denied ventilation, which would enhance their overall health and development, yet there is little hesitation in putting an adult on life support, even if he or she must then struggle for the "right to die."

"Perception" of ventilator dependency is another key factor. The words we use conjure images which shape attitudes and consequently behavior. What does "on" a ventilator actually mean? Is she lying, sitting, standing, or kneeling on it? Surely, to be accurate, the ventilator is on the person? Is it not more accurate to say the patient *uses* a ventilator? Or does she? Perhaps it is the health professional and not the patient?

Consider the word "patient." A patient is defined as someone who is dependent, acted upon, suffering, passive, ill. If an individual is perpetually cast in this role, he or she begins to behave accordingly. If, however, he or she is permitted to take charge of his or her life, to direct his or her own needs and function autonomously, the perception becomes that of a competent human who just happens to have unique physical characteristics which necessitate the use of specialized equipment in order to be able to function within his or her environment.

Consider the astronaut. He is dependent on complex assistive devices, even life support, in order to live and function in outer space, yet the astronaut is not perceived as defective, sick, or disabled. The astronaut is highly regarded in terms of competence and skill in managing and maintaining the equipment he is dependent upon. It is the environment which is considered aberrant and unable to meet his physiological needs.

Many ventilator users are "responauts." They are competent, responsible, and knowledgeable of their needs. They do not regard themselves as deficient or helpless. Rather, the environment with its physical, physiological, and attitudinal barriers is perceived to be the problem which challenges the attainment of personal autonomy and independence.

Personality and cognitive attributes are other key components. Psychologists talk about "hardiness" and its relationship to stress and illness. We know that stress correlates with a wide variety of illnesses and the immune system secretes fewer immunoglobins into the bloodstream when a person is under stress. We expect ventilator dependent persons to be sick more often, yet many actually become sick less often than the able-bodied. How can this be? Many long-term ventilator users are "hardy" people.

"Hardy" people handle stress well. They are survivors. They adapt to change and challenge by evaluating, diving in, and problem solving. They are responsible, active participants who take control and initiative in seeking solutions to stressful situations. They are not helpless observers. They look for a participatory relationship with health care providers and refuse to be victims. They educate themselves and become specialists in their own care because they want to share responsibility.

Bernie Seigal, in *Love, Medicine & Miracles*, describes such survivors as receptive, creative, and sometimes hostile, with a high degree of self-esteem. They are intelligent and self-reliant, with a strong sense of reality. They value interaction with others, of whom they are tolerant and concerned. They feel "empowered," in control of their lives and the systems they require to exist.

The Centre for Research in Education in Ontario, Canada, completed a two-year study of what "empowerment" is, how it happens, and what helps or hinders its development.

According to the study, no one factor creates a sense of powerlessness, but social isolation, segregation, and extremely low expectations by others are key contributors. Disconnectedness from the community, neighbors, peers, and family play a damaging role in perpetuating dependency and helplessness. In fact, some subjects defined their lives in terms of the demands, expectations, and direction of the services in their lives. They described how difficult it was to reframe their view of themselves as responsible citizens.

Empowerment almost always occurred when circumstances enabled an individual to develop a life in the community separate from their services. For some, service support was helpful in attaining this separateness. One-to-one support from a peer, a friend, or a service worker which was interactive, personalized, and mutually respectful was often the key to gaining a sense of control. "A good listener," "an equal," "a guide," "a person who really cares" were some of the adjectives used.

The process of empowerment often begins with a crisis, frustration, and outrage. Individuals discover they have a voice and that there are people who will listen. The inspiration and support of significant others as the individual carries out his or her desires, despite resistance or disapproval, matters enormously. There is a sense of control and choice, a critical awareness of the issues and opportunities for dialogue. A new sense of hope for the future occurs, a sense of being valued and nurtured by family, friends, society, service providers, and the community. Making connections with a network of similarly disabled peers who are knowledgeable and skilled in socio-political issues often provides the powerful bridge which takes a person from helplessness to action.

As the process of empowerment evolves, many people describe a growing confidence in their own capabilities and development of self-esteem. They describe an awareness that they too have "rights." The process of participating is self-empowering, as the social contacts initiated provide involvement in meaningful activity and reduce social isolation.

Autonomy derived from reality-based knowledge and experience, positive affirmation from those who provide support, strong cognitive and personal skills which enable a positive perception of the situation, and the empowerment which arises from strong social support are essential ingredients which enable many ventilator users to enjoy a worthwhile quality of life. Yet few professionals have knowledge or interest in such positivity. Why do we continue to focus on the tragic, costly, negative and hopeless images? Health care providers must gain knowledge of the entire spectrum of ventilator dependency. The positives must be balanced with the negatives. The real experts, ventilator users who have acquired skill and experience through several decades of dependency, are willing to share their secrets of life.

Hippocrates said, "It is better to know the patient who has the disease than it is to know the disease the patient has." If medicine can shift its organ-specific, failure-oriented approach to an approach which gives equal credence to the power of mind, spirit, and personality, then society's image of ventilator dependency need not be so narrow and dysfunctional.

REFERENCES

DeJong, G., "Defining and Implementing the Independent Living Concept," in N. Crwew and I. Zola, *Independent Living for Physically Disabled People*, 1983.

King, A.J., "Bridging the Gap Between ICU & Homecare: The Patient's Perspective." Keynote address (video presentation), 7th International Conference on Non-Invasive Ventilation, Orlando, Florida, March 1999.

_____, "Assessing Value, *Rehabilitation Digest*, 25(4), 1995:10–11.

_____, "Independent Living in the 90's," *Rehabilitation Gazette*, vol. 38(1), 1998.

_____, "Murder is Murder, Isn't It?" *Rehabilitation Digest*, vol.28(1/2), 1998: 14–16.

_____, (video), "A Patient's Perspective: From the ICU to Homecare," The CHEST Foundation, American College of Chest Physicians, Chicago, IL & American Asssociation for Respiratory Care, 1999.

_____, "Revisiting Rehabilitation: Some Thoughts on Control, Responsibility and Relationships, *Rehabilitation Digest*, vol. 27(3), 1997: 12–13.

_____, "Whose Life is it Anyway? Understanding Control, Responsibility and Patient/Physician Communication in Situations of Long Term Home Mechanical Ventilation," Meet-the-Professor Session, Proceedings of the 1998 conference of The American College of CHEST Physicians, Toronto, November 1998.

Lord, J., "Empowerment and Human Services: A Contradiction?" *Centre News Report*, 5:1, 1989.

Lord, J., et al., "Consumer Involvement," *Canada's Mental Health*, 37:2, 1989.

Seigel, B., *Love, Medicine & Miracles* (New York: Harper & Row, 1986).

Zola, I.K., "Healthism and Disabling Medicalization," in A. Illich, et al., ed., *Disabling Professions* (London, Marion Boyers, 1987).

9

DISCONTINUING VENTILATOR SUPPORT AT HOME

Clinical Experience with Amyotrophic Lateral Sclerosis in California

Barbara T. Beal, R.N., M.N.,
ALS Home Care Consultant

This chapter will review clinical experiences with individuals who had amyotrophic lateral sclerosis (ALS) and chose to discontinue ventilator breathing support.

Discussion includes an overview of the disease process; a brief discussion of persons who chose not to use life support devices; and the various roles the clinical nurse specialist played in the consultation process with this population. Case examples illustrate problems and approaches used with people dying of ALS.

THE DISEASE PROCESS

ALS is a devastating progressive motor neuron disease. It affects both upper and lower motor neurons controlling limb and bulbar muscle movement. Bladder and bowel sphincters, and other autonomic functions are not affected, nor are sexual, autonomic, or cardiac muscle functions. ALS can result in quadriplegia, loss of the ability to speak, swallow, and breathe, and eventuates in death. There is no known cause, treatment, prevention, or cure for ALS at the present time.

People who have ALS are usually cognitively intact adults; consequently they are able to take a primary role in making decisions regarding their own care and the optional life support systems required when vital functions are lost. A small number of my patients have shown cognitive incompetence. This seems to be representative of the estimated 5 percent of the adult onset "sporadic" form of the condition (1).

CLINICAL NURSE SPECIALIST ROLES

The clinical nurse specialist is a masters degree prepared person with roles including direct caregiver, teacher, researcher, advocate, and consultant. Functions as a home care consultant include all of these roles as patients, home settings, community resources, and family resources are evaluated. I provide teaching, consulting, referral, and liaison services, and direct the Orange County Support Group for ALS patients and families.

Services may also include counseling ALS patients and their families through a unique telephone consultation program sponsored by the Orange County Chapter of the ALS Association.

I have been directly involved with ten ALS clients in Orange County who, as they approached the endstage of the disease on life support, chose to discontinue the ventilator. Seven of them requested the medical director of the Muscular Dystrophy Association (MDA) of Orange County, Richard D. Dauben, M.D., to be the physician in attendance. With the legal consultant to the ALSA chapter, Dr. Dauben and I have developed the protocols described here.

FOCUS: EXPERIENCE WITH ENDSTAGE ALS

People with ALS eventually die. They hear about their prognoses from the physician who makes the diagnosis. Many are highly anxious and do not assimilate what their physician said unless time is spent to help them work through their anxieties.

It is clear that individuals with ALS think the thoughts discussed in this paper, even if they do not discuss them with anyone. There are many steps in the process of becoming aware, coping with disability and use of life support devices, facing death, and being ready to die. Some choose not to accept life support for breathing and eating, should these functions become paralyzed. Others choose to use life support devices. Some do not choose at all, but let events take their course. There is no right way.

In the United States, the latter choice seems to be the most common. This results in the physician deciding the course of action, usually during a predictable respiratory emergency. The critical factor brought to light by case examples here is that an informed decision-making process is critical, but not easy to obtain. To be assimilated, information has to be given at the level of the patient's understanding, at the time when he or she is psychologically ready to deal with it.

Many states do not permit patients to make decisions of the type under discussion. The patient's physician or someone else does. The current plethora of articles in professional and lay journals deals mostly with patients who are no longer capable of making choices. With ALS, only a rare few are unable to make decisions. Freedom of choice, however, is still relatively new, even in California, where the law does allow patient autonomy—providing the ground work is well laid.

TERMINAL ALS

Persons With No Life Support

Many fearsome stories are told and retold about strangling and choking as the way ALS patients die. In my experience, the stories are not true. But potent myths such as these create visceral responses that are nearly impossible to eradicate.

I have learned that people who are ready to die will do so quietly and peacefully. In a caseload of 250 over four years, I have identified 32 who requested a home consultation late in the disease stage and died shortly thereafter at home with no further medical treatment. When I have been privileged to be present, we were able to complete the necessary work without emotional trauma. All of the cases were variations of the following example.

Randolf F: Randolf's daughter Katherine called and asked for help because her father could not sleep. Randolf's speech was almost unintelligible, and his wife could not cope with his nursing needs due to her own severe medical problems. Katherine had taken leave from her job as a nursing home attendant to care for her father.

My initial visit was made at this point. I was able to phrase for him questions about oncoming breathing failure that he seemed unable to articulate, and told him how one dies with ALS.

Katherine telephoned me a month later to say that her father had had no more sleeping problems since my visit and had died peacefully. On the morning of his death, Katherine said, "It looks like today is the day, isn't it, Dad?" He smiled and agreed.

She arranged for his family and close friends to visit. As she bathed him in the afternoon, he became sleepy and died within the hour. He was rational to the end and did not choke.

The Ventilated Person

Some ALS patients choose to use ventilators prior to need. Some find themselves on ventilator life support without having chosen at all. However it occurs, one question remains uppermost in their minds: "I won't die of respiratory failure with a fatal neurological disease because I now have life support. But what will happen to me? How will I die?"

The answer is that the paralysis caused by the disease can continue until no voluntary muscles function, including eyelids. In practice, I have only seen one person who lived to this state. It is more common for ALS patients to die of untreatable intercurrent infections—usually pneumonias. Two individuals who had wanted life support no matter what happened died of circulatory insufficiency.

THE PROCESS

Close teamwork between the actors is essential. The team includes the patient, family, attorney, physician, home care nurse, and me.

A typical story can be told about a person with ALS going to the hospital with rapid onset respiratory failure, then becoming almost unresponsive. He wakes up to find himself mechanically ventilated and eventually is sent home on the ventilator. After a stormy adjustment and learning period, routines are established with caregivers around the clock.

The patient manages remarkably well and adjusts to the necessity of 24-hour care, suctioning, perhaps tube feedings, being turned every few hours and, frequently, being unable to speak.

Emotionally, there is devastation. He or she can do less for himself than before. There is an increasing lack of privacy and a feeling of being a useless burden. The patient is unable to express feelings. The time is passed by watching television and not thinking until the physical symptoms force attention to the unwanted thought, "I am really dying. Do I want to stay on this contraption forever?"

At this point, someone notifies one of the team.

Steps in the process of discontinuing life support are initiated. The steps take time—sometimes, several months. Whether the patient discusses it with the physician, keeps his thoughts private, or shares his thinking with a loved one, discontinuing life support is a topic which should be raised by the appropriate person—without fear of introducing an alien or aversive thought. Everyone on life support has thought about it at some time.

The issues to be addressed are fear, ignorance about what one's wishes really are, religious doctrine, and a natural repugnance to "managing" one's own death.

If the person is not ready to discuss it, there will be a natural turn-off point in the conversation. To the observant, sensitive onlooker, the person will signal when he or she is ready to talk.

ALS patients do not know what to expect. What may be clear to the professional is not known to the patient. Some do not know what questions to ask. They may fear what others may think, or what God thinks. Families may be surprized that their loved one has been thinking about dying at all because it is a taboo subject.

It is helpful if the professional involved in the care, frequently the nurse, be comfortable with his or her own thoughts about dying. Experienced nurses have usually faced spontaneous death many times. "Spontaneous" implies that no action was taken other than nursing care for a person who was not expected to survive.

Wish Identification

Frequently it is the home care nurse or a family member who identifies the ventilator-dependent person's wishes. They are in a position to have first-hand knowledge of the patient's motivation. The task, however, is complicated if the patient has become nonverbal from vocal cord paralysis.

When the home care nurse learns the patient's "readiness" motivation and wishes, she communicates them to the other members of the team.

Matthew. Matt has been on a ventilator for nine months. He is getting ready to set a date for discontinuing ventilation. A problem I anticipate is his being able to clarify his emotions.

Matt is a physicist whose life pattern is to make decisions mainly with the intellect. His voice is totally gone, his body paralyzed. He communicates with his big toe on an alphabet board. He has a great need to be in control, and is well-informed about his disease. He has excellent rapport with his physicians, who are willing to cooperate should he not wish to continue being ventilated. Because of their unfamiliarity with home disconnects, the physicians will want to admit Matt to the hospital at his bidding, should the occasion present itself.

Motivation Assessment

Evaluating what the motivation is, without outside influences, including the evaluators', is a delicate process. On the initial visit, I interview the person and ascertain his or her wishes and readiness to address the facts of the illness.

If the patient is ready, I outline exactly what is likely to occur, based on knowledge of human physiology and the process as we have experienced it. I am aware that the patient will use what I say to validate what he or she already knows.

Not uncommonly, the person is not yet ready to proceed. Time is needed to assimilate additional information. A second visit—in a month or more—can then be made.

Francis. At age 42, Francis had a rapid onset of ALS, requiring ventilator support only three months after his first symptom in December 1986.

He had not wanted any life support, but accepted it, since he was participating in an ALS clinical trial research program. To die before the research was finished could invalidate the data. Soon he realized that the research drug being administered was not helping him. He was getting worse. His desire to help science was mixed with his personal desire for healing.

I first visited Francis in April 1987. He and his wife, Shannon, had married when they were 16. She is a registered nurse. He wanted her to remove the ventilator but realized that she was not ready to let him die. He was also sensitive to her feelings, including possible future guilt.

Shannon felt that Francis was not ready to die, since he panicked whenever nursing help was not immediately available for his needs. (He had a chronic addiction to various tranquilizer medications.) Shannon received excellent support from her staff at work, including time off without loss of benefits, to be home with Francis. This helped her with the daily frustrations.

The necessary steps—legal, financial, and counseling—were initiated. I attended a care conference at the home health agency with the nurses and social worker. A lawyer arranged for a Durable Power of Attorney for Health Care (DPA/H). Francis chose not to take advantage of counseling referrals. Shannon became calmer as time went on.

In August, a physician agreed to admit Francis to a hospital and discontinue the ventilator. The physician did not permit himself to be made known and was uncomfortable providing this service in the home. Francis's death was peaceful. Three years later, Shannon continues to feel the right thing was done, in the best way possible.

Legal Process

There are few legal problems in California for the person wishing to withdraw artificial life support in the home.

A California Durable Power of Attorney for Health Care is used (2). Following signing, only witnesses or a notary public are needed to complete the document. If a patient cannot sign the paper or verbally indicate his or her wishes, a special addendum to the DPA/H has been developed.

We encourage use of a lawyer and notary when communication is totally compromised. It clarifies the decision making process for everyone. It can help to avoid later complications, should someone question whether the patient was coerced into "signing" his name. I use the version of the DPA/H devised by the California Medical Association, even though it includes items which may be considered extraneous to ALS patients, such as autopsy and body parts donation requests. The format of this version is recognized by most physicians as soon as they see it.

The process takes time.

Once the person has made up his or her mind, there is a tendency to want to rush things, to "Get on with the show." I do not encourage rushing. Impulsive decisions are often regretted. Assimilation time is vital for everyone's comfort level.

In the home, the choice is more private than it is in an institution. The person at home can choose and involve only those affected by the decision—the physician and health care team, family, and, if needed, the attorney.

Once the DPA/H is executed, copies should be given to all care providers who may need it—physician, hospital, home health agency, and family members.

Dialing 911

Calling 911 will invalidate the use of the California DPA/H. Dialing 911 is the equivalent of saying "rescue me." If the patient has opted for no life support and the attorney-in-fact notes that no life-prolonging measures are wanted, then two conflicting messages have been given at the same time—"let me die" and "save me." Paramedics who respond to the call must initiate resuscitation.

Some communities in California are working on policies that will allow paramedics to respond to 911 calls in such cases and honor the patient's wishes as expressed in the DPA/H.

No Code Orders

Where a professional from a home health agency is employed to care for an ALS patient, "Do Not Resuscitate" (DNR) or "No Code" orders must be written into the agency's chart before the planning for withdrawal of life support can be initiated. Otherwise, personnel would be obligated to resuscitate.

DNR orders are medical directives to home health agency personnel. Such orders mean that health care personnel are not obligated to resuscitate, perform heroics, or call 911 for paramedic help, should vital functions cease during endstage disease. The patient should be involved in the decision making, if capable of doing so.

Few home health agencies have policies at present, and there is no law covering the need for DNR orders in the home. They can be missed in day-to-day care planning. For most patients, this is not an emotional decision. It is usually clear in everyone's mind what is wanted; it has to be committed to paper only by the physician. By tradition, DNR orders are not accepted over the telephone. They must be written and signed personally by the physician before they are considered valid (3).

Contingency Planning for Arrests

Open communication leads to the next step: what to do in case of an emergency? This is best discussed after the patient is comfortable with the decision about the use of life support.

With no plan in place, a patient may be at the mercy of emergency room personnel to whom he or she is a stranger. They must perform treatments based on the policies and possible biases of the institution, which may be contrary to the patient's choice.

The contingency plan. By the telephone, or in a prominent place in the patient's home (not in a safe deposit box or the attorney's office), instructions should be available detailing exactly what to do in the event of a medical emergency, such as severe breathing difficulty. The instructions should include taking the DPA/H to the emergency room personnel. The attorney-in-fact under the power of attorney should be notified and available to state the patient's wishes.

Charlie Wedemeyer. A TV film special about Charlie Wedemeyer, football coach for the Los Gatos High School football team, showed that he wanted a ventilator when the need for one arose (4). His wife opposed the ER physicians, who never considered a ventilator as an option for an ALS victim.

Others clearly have not wanted life support yet have ended up on a ventilator because they could not, or did not, express their wishes when the time came.

Not to choose. Letting events decide for a patient is all right, and such a nonplan is a viable option. If the decision is difficult, nobody should be coerced into choosing, possibly creating intolerable anxiety.

The value of preplanning cannot be overstated. Interestingly, those who preplan seem to have fewer emergencies.

Physician Visit

When the first steps have been taken, a home visit is made by the attending physician to assess the patient's readiness to be taken off the ventilator, review the process again, meet and counsel the family, test the person off the ventilator, and set the date. As many family members as feasible should be present at this meeting.

Prescriptions

The family will fill any prescriptions for anxiety-relieving medications at the local pharmacy. There should be no problem with tablets which can be crushed for the feeding tube. Medication for injection is not a problem if ordered through the hospital pharmacy, where the physician is on staff.

Neighborhood pharmacies may be reluctant to fill prescriptions for one-time anti-anxiety injections.

I feel it is important that the family procure the medications. They are not dealing with an institution, where medication appears automatically, and filling the prescriptions helps clarify the family's readiness.

Discontinuing Ventilator Support

The home care nurse may be present when the patient is taken off the ventilator, depending on agency policy. This is encouraged, since terminal care is a special part of professional nursing practice and should not be denied a patient. It is not always possible, however, since many agencies in Southern California do not have a policy on the subject.

There are no reliable means of predicting how long a person on a ventilator can survive without it. Most people on ventilators are somewhat over-breathed. They have a mild "compensated respiratory alkalosis" and may breathe quite well for a short time after the ventilator is disconnected.

Sometimes a person survives weeks or months—when there is spontaneous breathing. This is unusual, in our experience. What usually happens is that no breaths are taken and we wait. Carbon dioxide alkalosis quietly turns into acidosis, and coma ensues. Soon, signs of life are gone. In ALS, there can be involuntary activity in small muscle groups for a short while, which should not be confused with signs of life or suffering.

Janet. Janet had been on life support for four years. She was accustomed to taking illicit drugs prior to the onset of ALS. She continually sought relief from pain, even when the pain was difficult to identify. While ALS does not result in pain, immobility can and does result in great discomfort.

Janet had, at one time, an implant portage system for morphine delivery to the paraspinal area for pain relief. This resulted in noncompliance with nursing efforts to turn her from side to side. She developed Stage 4 pressure sores that eroded from the bone of the lower spine.

When she finally asked to be taken off life support, Janet wanted total comfort. Fear was in her eyes when she addressed living on or dying. Nobody in her immediate environment could or would make the decision for her, although several visitors tried to persuade her to their point of view.

After the steps described above, which took six months to complete, the day came to remove the ventilator. Following several doses of anti-anxiety medication, she blinked out the words, "You promised me I'd be asleep and I'm not."

She had, of course, received no such promise. She indicated that she wanted to go ahead, but had exceeded the limits of the medication that could be prescribed safely without hospital admission. She was hospitalized and died quietly within minutes after the ventilator was removed, while receiving IV medication. Hospital policy was supportive, as their bioethics committee had clear guidelines in place after experience with previous ALS cases.

One cannot completely tag the experience as peaceful, even though there was no physical struggle. Her case illustrates the difficulty that we in a "free" society can have if we avoid the life experience of making a decision for which we alone are responsible.

Making a decision such as this was almost too much for Janet, but nobody let her "off the hook," and she did make the decision. A one-year follow-up call was made to her mother, who expressed her being at peace about Janet's decision, although she did need reassurance that there had been no physical struggle.

The following case is an example of someone who was totally at peace with his decision and relatively free of anxiety.

Pepe. Pepe had been a paraplegic due to polio prior to his quadriplegia from ALS. He had four years on a ventilator and survived several bouts with pneumonia.

He had a habit of meditating and praying at 1:00 daily, when all nursing activity ceased for an hour. When he requested my first visit to help him prepare for going off the ventilator, he was calm and straightforward within his nonverbal comments and responses to my questions.

He had had regular discussions with his priest, who was supportive, whatever decision Pepe made. A physician was quick to provide verbal orders for him to be taken off the ventilator by the nurse on duty—even before he had met the patient. The family was upset and the nurse rightly refused to obey the orders.

Discontinuance of a medical treatment with life-and-death consequences is not a traditional nursing responsibility in the home, so the consulting neurologist was invited to the home. He had known Pepe through MDA support services and a previous home visit. Pepe accepted anti-anxiety medication even though he was totally peaceful.

His wife, five children, nurse, priest, and I gathered around Pepe's bed. I suggested to him that he was taking a medication, not his custom, for his family's anxiety—not for his own. He grinned and nodded.

Over 200 people attended his funeral. The priest discussed Pepe's decision in his remarks. Many friends and family commented afterwards on the sense of celebration of a life well lived.

FOLLOW-UP

Several months after death, I normally call the family member who was closest to the ALS patient. This is valuable for them and for me. I try to clarify any confusion and provide emotional support, which seems to be appreciated. I have yet to meet regret or "second thoughts" in my patients' families. I attribute this to the discipline of carefully following the readiness steps outlined in this paper, and to open communication between the patient, the team, and the family.

COMMENTS

Discontinuing Ventilators—From Reluctance to Alacrity?

Physicians' attitudes seem to be changing as legal safeguards are followed and become accepted. With laws and sanctions in place, as in California, there will come a time when the physician who choses *not* to comply with a person's wishes will be more vulnerable than those who do.

Then we may well have to deal with another problem that Eva's experience demonstrates: physicians who will discontinue life support with too much alacrity—before the patient and family have had time to adapt to the decision and its consequences. Safeguards must be established—perhaps best through the work of hospital and home health agency bioethics committees.

Eva: Eva was going downhill with ALS. She could not make up her mind about life support. She was starving and had less than 1 liter forced vital capacity (FVC) when tested the previous year. She had not been tested since. She did sign a DPA/H, opting for all life support unless she was in irreversible coma. She made no other plans, nor did her home care staff know her wishes.

During an incident, Eva was hospitalized at the nearest medical facility and eventually placed on life support, but not before she lapsed into an irreversible coma. The attorney-in-fact stated that Eva's wishes were to discontinue use of a ventilator if she went into a coma. A neurological examination was done, and a conference was held in the physician's office with the nursing consultant, attorney, hospital physician, and two of her children. A third son was asked to wait in the reception room.

The doctor responded to the patient's legally prepared request with such alacrity that there was insufficient time for the entire family to be involved. After a risk assessment by an infection control nurse, Eva was taken off the ventilator following a physician phone order to the unit nurses.

At the time of Eva's death, her sister was enroute from Israel.

I informed the family about the "weaning" being initiated. They left the hospital thinking she looked nearly normal. Eva died shortly after they arrived back at the hospital. During a follow-up home visit, Eva's sister expressed a fatalistic acceptance of what could not be helped.

Questions raised: Compassion by the physician is mandated by the Hippocratic oath, but this does not insure physician objectivity. A third party payor, almost by definition, will be interested in shortening its fiscal responsibility. Families need time to work through their feelings about having the person alive or letting them die. Any one of us can have prejudice about who is valuable to society and who is not. Can bioethics committees serve this function? Will physicians guard their honor from within? Will families be counseled so they can disengage themselves from their grief and biases?

Until these questions are addressed, we should be hesitant to respond too quickly, just as we now tend to respond too slowly after a person has cried "enough." This is a human, humane, soul searching, and mind searching time for people in a free society.

We in the United States say we value individual autonomy. We must allow ourselves the space to mature in wisdom so we can grow up to the responsibility.

NEED FOR PROFESSIONAL INVOLVEMENT

One could ask why professionals need to be involved at all—especially when the person is at home. Why not just "pull the plug"? This has been done. Aside from the moral or religious issues, it can be legally complicated.

A coroner's inquest is required for any unexplained death in the US. Publicity is likely to follow. The secrecy required is akin to planning a suicide, and the stress is unnecessary where due process of law includes the right to decline further medical treatment.

CONCLUSION

In my opinion, the most important part of the process of ending home ventilation of a patient is ascertaining and accepting the patient's wishes, whatever they may be. There is a peaceful air about a person who is sure and who has made his or her decision. There are no more tears. If smiles can be beatific, this is when we see them. When everything seems to come together, I concur with so many of my families that the death of their loved one was "a celebration of life."

NOTES

1. Tandan, Rup, "Amyotrophic Lateral Sclerosis: Part 1. Clinical Features, Pathology and Ethical Issues in Management," *Annals of Neurology* 1985, 18:271–280.

2. California Medical Association, Durable Power of Attorney for Health Care Form, revised, 1989. This document follows the California Civil Code #2420-2443 (or #2500 et. seq.).

3. Tennenhouse, Dan J., "NO-CODE ORDERS," *California Nurses Digest*, August 1986, vol. 52.

4. "One More Season," video film for television on the life of Charlie Wedemeyer, Crystal Bullet Productions, 1989. Distrib. by Bridgestone Group.

REFERENCES

Beal, Barbara T. "Breathing Failure in ALS and Handling Emergencies." *Reaching Out, Newsletter for the ALS Association, Orange County Chapter,* Oct./Nov., 1989.

Beal, Barbara T. "Life Support: Is it for You?" *Reaching Out, Newsletter for the ALS Association, Orange County Chapter,* Aug./Sept., 1990.

Goldblatt, David. "Decisions about Life Support in Amyotrophic Lateral Sclerosis." *Seminars in Neurology,* 1984, 4:1:104–110.

Holden, Dee. *Thoughts on Decision Making for Ventilators.* San Francisco: ALS and Neuromuscular Research Foundation, 1986.

LeMaistre, JoAnn. *Beyond Rage: How to Cope with Emotional Problems of Chronic Physical Illness.* Oak Park, IL, PO Box 183, 90303: Alpine Guild, 1985.

McLeod, Don." Matter of Life and Death: Supreme Court Soon Will Rule on Who Can Decide." *AARP,* 1990, 7–8.

"Questioning Autonomy in Health Care Decision Making." *Ethical Currents.* Center for Bioethics, St. Joseph Health System and California Association of Catholic Hospitals, Nov. 1986, No. 9.

Ross, J., et al. "A Process for Resolving Bioethical Dilemmas." *Handbook for Hospital Ethics Committees.* AHA: 1986.

Ruark, John E., and Thomas Alfred Raffin. "Initiating and Withdrawing Life Support." *NEJM,* 1988, 318:25–30.

Sebring, Deborah L., and Paul Moglia. "Amyotrophic Lateral Sclerosis: Psychological Interventions for Patients and Their Families." *Health and Social Work,* Spring 1987, 114–120.

Tamborlane, Theodosia A. "A Patient's Right to Refuse or Discontinue Treatment." *Caring,* 1987, 30–31.

Tandan, Rup, and Walter G. Bradley. "Amyotrophic Lateral Sclerosis: Part 1. Clinical Features, Pathology and Ethical Issues in Management." *Annals of Neurology*, 1985, 8:272, 1985.

Wanzer, Sidney H., et al. "The Physician's Responsibility Toward Hopelessly Ill Patients." *NEJM*, 1989, 320:844–9.

10

DESCRIPTION OF SELF

Albert Anderson

Tubes come from or enter my orifices
And I begin to seek reasons for my existence.
I continue to be
In spite of—not because.

The pulmonary cripple, particularly with a progressive neurological disorder, is totally dependent—a disaster, climbing, figuratively, on a lattice work of humanity. (This may disappear at any moment.) If the supporting lattice works well, it calls to mind a young Englishman's comment on Americans and American TV programs on disability. He said wryly, "when you hear Americans talking about the disabled, you almost hear them say with a certain glee . . . 'paraplegia must be fun.'"

When we talk about total dependency, there is no privacy. You are moved from one machine to another. You whine, you complain. Your very life depends on a tube. You can't make a phone call without assistance.

God, why me?
BECAUSE, IT IS YOUR TURN.

A fever of activity is my coping mechanism. I am made mobile by a wheelchair Bantam Ventilator, although I sleep with an Emerson ventilator.

Depression comes early in the morning, just after awakening. I spend my time coughing and spitting. I seldom sleep. I live with fear, anger, and resentment. My nurse says I am a wimp.

LONELINESS

Loneliness goes with my chronic disease.
A quiet separation from the outside world occurs
from other people, from places, from things.
At first its presence devastated me,
But this settled down to a quiet emptiness
That permeated each moment of my life.
Visitors and acquaintances marvel at my bravery
In my dealings with affliction,
But they cannot enter my world of unrelenting discomfort.
Contact with others does not dispel this sense of loneliness.
It is a miasma that spreads to those about me
And they too feel cut off, lonely.
Sometimes I think, "If I could fly,"
But even this would be a solitary action.

Is there no room for others in this shell of self-indulgence?
I withdrew slowly from the real world.
I am not sure who withdrew from whom,
But the separation occurred.
Real life moves so fast,
The train has no room for a car with rusty wheels.
I show flashes of life
And make occasional ineffective thrusts at the world,
But I quickly settle back to contemplate my personal needs.
Not that I lack for carers,
But these are strange hands for such intimacy.
But strangers must care for me,
Lest I add an additional burden to my loved ones.
Oh, how I miss those warm, knowing hands.

And then you have to get used to pills, euphemistically called rotation of medication.

11

ETHICAL ISSUES RELATED TO THE SPECIAL CARE UNIT

Barbara J. Daly, R.N., M.S.N., F.A.A.N.

Our original purpose in opening the Nurse Managed Special Care Unit (SCU) was two-fold: to improve the care delivery for a particular group of patients, the chronically, critically ill, and to increase the job satisfaction of registered nurses. The essential differences between the care delivered in the SCU and that provided in traditional intensive care units (ICUs) are the environment and the focus of care. Unlike ICUs, the environment of the SCU is not designed to isolate the patient and concentrate large amounts of technologically sophisticated resources on curing a pathological condition (which is an effective way of getting a patient through a short-term crisis). Instead, our emphasis is on demedicalizing the total illness experience, which is viewed not as an episode, but as a phase in the life of the person. The focus is on providing care for the entire person, in the fullest meaning of that word. While we hope to facilitate the passage through this illness phase to a more functional, comfortable phase of life, and we do use some fairly complex treatment regimens in order to do this, the interventions are the tools, not the focus of our interactions.

To measure the effectiveness of this approach, we designed an experimental research program, which consists of random assignment of patients to the experimental group (and transfer to the SCU) or to the control group (who remain in the traditional ICU) and the measurement of objective outcomes, such as LOS, cost, mortality, and complication rates. In addition, we measure patient and family satisfaction, using standard tests which meet the usual psychometric criteria. Our experience to date has clearly indicated that the SCU unit is a success. Patients and families repeatedly express satisfaction with getting out of the high-tech environment of the ICU and appreciate the more comfortable, "user-friendly" atmosphere of the SCU. The cost and mortality data clearly indicate that we are able to achieve the same outcomes with significantly lower costs. These represent the hoped-for positive results.

However, we did *not* expect the effect of taking this group of patients out of the ICUs and grouping them together in one place, which has allowed us to see more clearly what is characteristic about them as a group. By having them together in one unit, patterns and similarities that were less evident when they were "mixed" among the traditional ICU population have become clear and have presented us with a whole new set of questions about what we *are* doing for these people, what we *can* do, and what we *should* do.

WHAT WE ARE DOING

Look for a moment at the discharge outcomes for the first 30 patients (Table 1). A little less than one-third of the total group (experimental plus control) went home, another third (11) died, and the final one-third went to some type of extended care facility. It is the last two groups that I will describe.

TABLE 1. Discharge Outcomes

OUTCOME	EXPERIMENTAL	CONTROL	TOTAL
Home	5	3	8 (28%)
Nursing Home	3	5	8
Rehab. Facility	2	0	2 10 (39%)
Died	6	3	9 (32%)

First, consider the patients in an extended care facility. The characteristics of this group are not surprising. They are generally older (65 to 80 years of age); all have some degree of chronic illness (primarily diabetes, left ventricular failure, COPD, and neurological deficit, such as stroke); all have lost considerable functional ability during hospitalization; and the great majority are still capable of recovering some of this function at the point of being ready to be discharged from the acute care setting. The problem we face is that there is no facility designed to meet their continuing care needs. These are, by and large, people who cannot go home for a variety of reasons: their care is too complex to be managed easily at home (e.g., requiring IV antibiotics via Broviac catheter, tube feedings, physical therapy, etc.), there is no family to help at home, or they cannot afford the amount of professional home care that would be necessary. However, it is clear to us that continued slow, gradual work to increase their level of independence, further their ability to feed themselves, and accomplish other activities of daily living (with attention to the psychological aspects of recovering from a state of total dependency and life-threatening illness) will increase their functional level. This, in some cases, would eventually lead to their being able to go to their own home or the home of a relative. Unfortunately, there do not seem to be any facilities which provide this "in-between" care—a level of care "in between" a nursing home and a rehabilitation facility. The patients in this group are unable to take part in most rehabilitation programs—they are too frail to tolerate the six hours of active therapy that a rehabilitation facility must provide in order to get reimbursed at rehabilitation and not the lower nursing home rates; yet, traditional nursing homes are not designed to focus on rehabilitation.

This problem has two components. First, the operational difficulty of finding placement for these patients. It is very tempting to keep them in the hospital, where they will get some rehabilitation and continue to make some gains in functional ability. This is obviously a poor second-best, however. Aside from the expense involved, acute care hospitals are not really good at rehabilitation. The alternative, however, is to send the patient to a nursing home, knowing that by doing so he or she will most likely not improve any further.

The second, equally serious problem, is justifying bringing a patient this far, knowing that there is no place to go if we succeed in getting them through the initial crisis. The average hospital cost (not bill, actual cost) of this phase of care is $100,000, which does not take into account the effort, stress, and suffering these patients and their families endure during the average six-week stay in the hospital. The subset of this group that illustrates this problem even more clearly is the few patients who become ventilator dependent for life. If their families are unable to care for them physically or financially, these people truly have no place to go. In our geographic area, there is only one facility that will take ventilator dependent patients on Medicare, and it has a two-year waiting list. The options of patients in this group come down to three: remain in the acute care hospital; wait for a bed in that one facility, or elect to be terminally weaned from ventilatory support.

By taking the patients in this group out of several ICUs, keeping them together rather than transferring them to different general divisions, and having the same social worker, physician, and nurses make discharge plans for them, we have a different view of what technology has created, a side effect of success. We are beginning to come to grips with the implications of this issue; there is no question, however, that we must rethink our mission with these patients.

Of the patients who died, only two were unexpected arrests. In the other cases, a decision was made either to stop therapy or withdraw therapy. This, too, is a situation familiar to ICU personnel. Because it is so common to our group, however (having occurred in almost 30 percent of the cases), it has both immediate implications for care and long-range implications for how hospitals are managed.

WHAT WE SHOULD DO

One of the effects of the above is to underscore that it is imperative to immediately address the patient's wishes regarding resuscitation. This is not always easy, nor is it appreciated at the time. These people did not think they had a terminal illness; they had an acute event. Most of them were very functional, living independently at home. Half of them only came to the hospital to have surgery. They have spent weeks in an environment that is dedicated to saving life and curing, and now we introduce the subject of DNR status and limits to how much more we invest.

The second clear need is to become more knowledgeable about "terminal weaning," an irreversible plan of progressive weaning from ventilatory support, knowing this will in all likelihood lead to death. This is not new to critical care, but it is a subject that is being brought "out of the closet," enabling us to learn how to handle it in a more skillful and humane fashion. For example, we have learned that there are five distinct phases prior to initiating weaning: explanation, reassurance, a "cooling off" period, mobilization of support resources, and the exact timing of the weaning.

Explanation is crucial. If the option of weaning is explained properly, it enables patients and their families to a see it as a real choice, rather than one of the inevitable phases of hopelessness, suicide, or even murder. The option of removing ventilatory support is presented the same way as the choice of refraining from surgery, for example—a choice made according to what they want from life and how they want to live it, given the unalterable facts of their illness or condition. Repeated reassurance that we will not let the patient suffer pain or gasp for breath, and that there will be time to think things over, is necessary. When we first discuss this issue, we repeatedly state that the procedure can be aborted at any step, if the patient or family change their minds.

The cooling-off period is very important. Many families struggle with this decision and come to a consensus, only to change their minds. Allowing a day between the decision and beginning the wean allows for quiet deliberation.

We are accustomed to providing support resources for families in crisis, and this situation requires them. Importantly, different types of support are sometimes needed at two distinct times—one, to help make the decision (this is often our Hospital Ethics Committee or the patient's minister) and another support figure to be with the family during the weaning period. This is usually other family members or close friends. Our job, of course, is to investigate who can be helpful and make whatever arrangements we can to get the supports there at the right time.

The timing of all of this is difficult to judge, as is usually the case with decisions regarding life support withdrawal. For the time to be right, we need three things. The caregivers have to have time to gather sufficient information about the diagnosis and prognosis and get to know the patient and the family, in order to evaluate their emotional and physical status. The patient, if awake, has to have enough time to think through the decision. The family needs time, too. Obviously, this is a very individual element, but it would be helpful to have some general signposts which could be used in developing a plan.

There are no textbooks, studies, or lessons available to tell us how to do this. Taking people off ventilators is done every day in American hospitals, but our ambivalence about it has prevented the careful study we would ordinarily do to learn the hows and whens. We have a general outline, which directs caregivers about the steps and the order of the steps to be taken, but we don't know, for example, how rapidly these steps should be taken, which step should come first, whether it is necessary to sedate a patient to the level of no response to pain in order to be certain he or she is not experiencing a shortness of breath. We also do not have data regarding whether patients who are conscious but sedated perceive hunger if we do not feed them. In thinking about these questions, the moral issues must be considered. Another way to describe this subset of patients, which highlights the moral issues, is to think of them as people who cannot live outside the ICU. Their disease is advanced, and treatment is complex and very resource intensive. By keeping them in the ICU or the SCU, we can keep them alive; sending them to a less intensive facility inevitably results in life-threatening deterioration. Some of these patients decide to stop, and those are the ones just described. Some go to a nursing home, only to die within two or three weeks. In a few cases, the patient chooses treatment when we raise DNR issues.

These last patients force us to confront the question of what we should do. We *are* providing care, sometimes cure, at a more cost-effective (albeit still quite expensive) rate for this population of very sick, elderly people. We know that we can respond to a patient's wish to stop treatment and remove technological support in a comfortable, caring fashion. What we do not know is what we *should* do, in the long run, for patients such as these. We probably all agree to a general level of imperative, such as we can not afford to offer everything to everyone. But what does this mean on an individual hospital level? Should we have three types of ICUs—the traditional hyperaggressive treatment unit, a unit like our SCU for the more long-term, less aggressive focus, and perhaps an ICU-hospice type of unit, where patients can be even more comfortably and less expensively cared for? If we know, for example, when we send Mr. Smith to a nursing home, where he will no longer receive our precise fine-tuning of his left ventricular failure and will not be suctioned every two hours, that he will be in the group which dies within a week or two. Would it not be better to have a facility within the hospital, a hospice environment, where Mr. Smith could go?

And what of Mr. Brown, who has been with us for three months and continues to want all interventions? If we confront the fact that we cannot afford to keep him in the ICU for the rest of his life, which could be months, should we define this before we start treatment or at least in the early phases of treatment, so we can tell him that this will not be an option, that ICU resources cannot be used for more than *x* number of months, that his choices cannot include continued readmission to the ICU?

These questions are not new, but they have been brought into focus by our work in the Special Care Unit. We believe that our technological successes will continue and that this will inevitably result in more patients reaching chronic critical illness. It is essential that we aggressively develop guidelines that will assist us and our patients in facing the difficult moral and economic challenges presented.

12

CASE HISTORY REPORT—THE ATYPICAL PATIENT

An Adolescent with ALS in an ICU

Marilyn M. Rawnsley, D.N.Sc.

Special hospital units develop distinctive cultures. Although embedded in a larger context of administrative and medical mores, the units are distinguished by the specificity of their services and skills, their self-restricted group identity, and the common characteristics of their patients. Changes in any of these dimensions may disturb the accustomed rhythms of the milieu. Occasionally, if a disruption is severe or too rapid or too encompassing, administrative assistance—as foresight or hindsight—may be required to restore equilibrium. But in most circumstances, for example, expansion or delegation of skills, additions or attritions to staff, increase in patient acuity and introduction of new technology, there is a self-limiting phase of transitional instability as the changes are assimilated into the unit culture.

There is, however, one cultural anomaly observed by this author and verified by other clinicians which appears to lie outside the cultural adaptation zone of many special units. This aberrant phenomenon is the admission of the atypical patient. For the purposes of this chapter, an atypical patient is defined as one whose characteristics and needs are perceived by the staff to lie outside their range of expertise. Whether or not the perception is accurate is not the issue. This chapter reports on the admission of one atypical patient to an intensive care unit, in which outside assistance was sought, and discusses that clinical illustration in terms of its general clinical relevance.

CASE HISTORY

The patient, a 19-year-old male, was admitted to the intensive care unit through the emergency room of a 300-bed community hospital in a suburban area 30 miles outside of a major Northeastern city. One year earlier, the patient had been diagnosed as having Amyotrophic Lateral Sclerosis (ALS), and until ten days prior to admission, he had been receiving treatment at a major medical center in the city. Since all efforts, including experimental therapies, had not slowed the rapidly progressing disease process, the patient had returned home in the care of his mother. He was unknown at the community hospital and to the attending physician. An area neurologist who had accepted the referral from the medical center was scheduled to see the patient later that week.

According to the emergency room physician's note, the patient arrived by ambulance in acute respiratory distress, accompanied by his mother, who was reported as stating that she did not want any extraordinary measures taken to prolong his life. The E.R. physician apprised the attending neurologist by telephone of the circumstances and requested that he come immediately to the hospital. The neurologist declined, but reportedly responded, "I wouldn't intubate him if I were you." The E.R. physician nevertheless intubated the patient and admitted him to the ICU, the only unit in the hospital that could provide the necessary technological care for a patient on a ventilator.

Within 24 hours, the patient's condition stabilized, and within a few days the head nurse of the ICU requested a meeting with the psychiatric nurse consultant, who was available to staff on an hourly basis. In itself, this request signaled unusual distress, since the nurse consultant service had been established for over a year but had never been called. The meeting took place on the unit, with most of the day staff and representatives from the evening and night staffs present. The nurses had called the consultant to verify the inappropriateness of this patient for the ICU and to intercede with administration and hasten his transfer to another institution. The request for transfer had already been made, but social service had advised the staff that there were few long-term facilities able to care for patients on ventilators and the waiting period could be three or four weeks or more. The staff, well respected for their calm, efficient competence, was visibly distraught. The only solution they could see was the removal of this inappropriate patient from their unit.

The consultant took advantage of the hour set aside for the conference to explore the situation, gathering data and suggesting a plan "to help them through the waiting period." Since the problem was the nursing staff's distress (the patient's medical condition was stable), the consultant focused on discussion of the recurring theme in their complaints, the admission itself. The emergency room physician was the immediate target of their anger. Why did he intubate the patient? Initially, the neurologist, one of "their group," was spared. As the discussion progressed, the nurses stopped defending him and expressed resentment that he had not protected them from this traumatic experience. Later, they expressed disappointment that he had not lived up to their expectations and taken charge in the emergency room. Eventually, one nurse admitted anger at the patient's mother for giving mixed messages: bringing him to the E.R. and then not wanting him to be treated. This admission refocused the discussion on the patient's mother, and general anger surfaced, not only because of her emergency room behavior, but also because she had not been back to visit the patient since admission. The staff, which took pride in its crisis skills, perceived this potentially long-term patient to have been "dumped" on them, first by his mother, then by the physicians, and finally by an unresponsive administration.

Since there was not much time left, and no one had talked about the patient, the consultant asked the staff to describe him to her. The group mood shifted from righteous anger to hushed hesitancy. The patient was described as a late adolescent, extremely thin, unable to move except to blink his eyes and to press the call bell with his right index finger, something he did whenever a nurse was not in his room. He was conscious but devoid of expression except for his eyes, which the staff interpreted as anxious and frightened. Since he required total care, his basic nursing was assigned to two senior nursing students; staff nurses handled only his complex technical care (i.e., ventilator care). The rationale was that the nursing students needed the experience and the staff was freed to attend to its critically ill—or typical—patients.

Although a detailed account of the processes by which the consultant helped the staff to move beyond its distress to that of the patient is germane to understanding motion towards empathy for another through the medium of self-empathy, the brevity of this report suggests that focus as the subject for another paper. For the purpose of this case illustration, only a summary of the outcome is included.

OUTCOME SUMMARY

Several conferences were scheduled to implement the plan, evaluate progress, and offer support, guidance, and when necessary, redirection.

1. The head nurse called the patient's mother to advise her of the patient's condition, offer support, and encourage her to visit the patient when she was ready. The patient's mother revealed that her husband had died in an accident shortly before their son was diagnosed with ALS. Although she understood that her son had returned home from the medical center to die, she had panicked when he went into respiratory distress and did not want to be alone with him when he died. She was embarrassed, and angry with

herself for bringing him to the hospital. She accepted the staff's support and began to visit her son regularly. The staff tried to arrange time to speak with her on each visit.

2. While his mother was being contacted, a designated member of the nursing staff "talked" to the patient in an attempt to explain his mother's absence. The nurse told the patient that if she were he, she would be wondering what happened to her mother. The nurse told him that his mother was very tired, that she would be in to see him when she could, and that she loved him very much. When asked if he understood, the patient blinked his eyes twice for "yes." Subsequently, the continuous ringing of the call bell diminished.

3. Staff nurses in the ICU assumed responsibility for the patient's basic physical care, with assistance from a senior nursing student. Personal care was given by an experienced nurse, based on the hypothesis that the nursing student, being a peer of the patient, might be a source of embarrassment to him.

4. Since the patient was in a room by himself, the staff were encouraged to "humanize" the environment. Halloween was approaching, and the staff decorated his room accordingly.

5. The head nurse of the ICU spoke with the neurologist about the purpose and content of the staff conferences and invited him to attend. He did not, but began to talk with the staff about the patient and to support its efforts.

6. After two weeks, the staff thanked the consultant and told her they would call her if they needed her again. They had regrouped, and no longer needed outside intervention. They also told her that they had advised social service there was no urgency to transfer the patient. Six weeks later, the patient expired on the intensive care unit.

DISCUSSION

This case report of an intensive care unit nursing staff's response to what it perceived as an inappropriate admission illustrates a number of the issues generated by the cultural anomaly of the atypical patient. Labeling the patient "inappropriate" set up a mechanism for rejection; the staff felt justified in perceiving the patient's needs as outside the scope of its expertise and thus drawing its energies from the patients who could benefit from its special skills. The labeling of patients is not unique to intensive care units. Consider the psychotic patient on a surgical floor; the patient on the psychiatric unit whose medical condition requires monitoring and intervention; the adult patient assigned to an empty pediatric bed due to medical overflow; or the terminal cirrhosis patient on an oncology unit. The issue of atypical patients who violate the cultural norm may be so common that the insidious effects on staff function and morale are overlooked.

The disorganization of staff, manifested in looking for a scapegoat, resentment, and hostility, must be recognized and addressed in order to minimize breakdown in staff communication and cohesiveness, which may result in emotional isolation from the patient and a distortion of the patient's needs. The energy mobilized to have the patient removed from the unit can be redirected towards helping the staff members widen their cultural adaptation zone to include the atypical patient. Of course, this approach is based on a careful assessment of the staff's perception; if the real issue is patient safety, then other measures must be implemented.

In the case presented, several factors contributed to the positive outcome. Most notable were the early recognition of the problem by the nursing staff, the request for consultation (though the motive was to have the problem removed), the availability of a nursing consultant, and the crisis orientation of the staff which was conducive to reframing the problem. What was most successful was the shift in focus from the wishful "what ifs" to the pragmatic "what now." When the reality is terminal illness, the importance of confronting "the here and now" seems the only reasonable approach.

13

USE OF LONG-TERM ASSISTED MECHANICAL VENTILATION IN PATIENTS WITH SPINAL MUSCULAR ATROPHY

Irene S. Gilgoff, M.D.
Emily Kahlstrom, M.D.
Eithne MacLaughlin, M.D.
Thomas G. Keens, M.D.

The use of long-term assisted mechanical ventilation continues to gain acceptance in patients with neuromuscular disease. Reports of patients with Duchenne's muscular dystrophy (1) using life support equipment have increased in the literature. Varying types of assisted ventilation have been used, including negative pressure machines (2) such as the iron lung and body wrap, competing with positive pressure devices such as tracheal (3), mouth (1), and now nasal (4) positive pressure systems. Reports of varying success of long-term ventilation in children with mixed neuromuscular diagnoses (5) led us to review the data we had gathered on all children diagnosed with spinal muscular atrophy (SMA) that we had treated with assisted ventilation (6). The study consisted of a retrospective chart review. It was a joint effort of three major Los Angeles area hospitals that care for children: Rancho Los Amigos Medical Center, Childrens Hospital Los Angeles, and the Los Angeles County-University of Southern California Medical Center.

A review of the charts yielded 15 children with SMA who had been placed on assisted ventilation. The group included two children we classified as having the severe Werdnig-Hoffmann form of the disease, with the remaining 13 having the intermediate form. The two patients with severe SMA had slightly varying courses. One child required assisted ventilation as early as five months of age. From this early age, he had severe facial and bulbar involvement. The second patient (and a third child that we have ventilated since completion of the study) had severe involvement of all four extremities, the trunk, and the respiratory muscles, all within the first few months of life. She was not able to sit unassisted. Her cough and voice were weak. Bulbar muscles were involved. She did not, however, require assisted ventilation until 15 months of age. Although she did not as easily fit the classical presentation, where respiratory failure occurs within the first six months to one year of life, her course was markedly different from the 13 other children in the study. The 13 other patients, felt to be classical of the intermediate form of the disease, did not require mechanical assisted ventilation until older, with a range of from 9 years 4 months to 17 years 7 months, the average being 14 years.

Our goals in treatment of all 15 of the patients were twofold. The first goal was educating the family and the patient (if old enough) about the alternative of assisted ventilation. This education process made the family an active participant and a guiding factor in the treatment program. The second goal was early prediction of respiratory compromise, with subsequent planned intervention. These goals were the same goals that we had with our DMD patients, yet we quickly found that predictability with DMD was a much easier task than it was in our patient population with SMA. In DMD, decline of pulmonary function is easily assessed by the gradual and progressive fall in the forced vital capacity (FVC)(7). A FVC of 500 ccs. heralded respiratory failure usually within six months to one year. The onset of CO_2 retention was a clear and ominous hallmark of impending respiratory failure (7). With so predictable a course, an organized program for family and patient education was relatively easy to establish. Options of using a ventilator or respecting the natural progression of the disease could be presented early and dealt with slowly and repeatedly, so decisions could be made without the additional pressure of an emergency medical situation.

From the standpoint of predictability, SMA, however, is a much more difficult disease to treat than DMD (6). FVC values did not prove to be useful in predicting when the chronic respiratory muscle weakness would progress to acute respiratory failure. CO_2 retention was also not a helpful predictor. In contrast, we found that most of our patients with SMA ran chronically low CO_2s. In the SMA patient, hypocapnea was the normal state. Instead, hypoxia was the first sign of respiratory compromise.

The roots of the differences in the presentation of respiratory failure between DMD and SMA go to the roots of pediatrics and to one of pediatrics' unique aspects—that of growth and development. In DMD, respiratory failure occurs during adolescence. A chest x-ray of an adolescent with DMD reveals little to no difference from the chest x-ray of a normal child. The intercostal muscles, still strong in early childhood, have shaped a normal chest wall that encompasses the child's normal lungs. By the time respiratory failure becomes imminent, chest wall integrity has been firmly established.

In SMA, this is not true. Instead, weakness of the intercostal muscles is an early hallmark of the disease. As growth occurs, the rib cage is pulled down—controlled by the downward pull of the diaphragm. This occurs due to the absence of the normal action of the intercostal muscles (8). The chest of a young child with SMA reveals complete loss of integrity of the chest wall. The continuing pull of the diaphragm downward—lacking the opposing forces of the intercostals—actually encourages lung collapse.

The dynamics of the chest wall explain the difference in the presentation of respiratory failure in children with SMA. Clinically, such children breathe with rapid shallow breaths throughout their lives, to minimize diaphragm movement and the inevitable stress it places on the chest wall. The rapid respiratory rate accounts for the low CO_2s seen. When the child gets an upper respiratory infection or pneumonia and deeper breaths are required, lung collapse becomes increasingly common due to the lack of intercostal muscle strength. The lung collapses and shunting occurs. Hypoxia follows.

The child with SMA is set up for this sequence of events for an additional reason, which also deals with the pattern of muscle weakness classical to this disease and occurring from a very early age. The second influence is the severe weakness of the abdominal muscles inherent to SMA. Without strong abdominal muscles, the patient is unable to cough effectively (9). This failed ability to clear the upper respiratory system of secretions again sets the patient up for infections of the lower respiratory tract.

Consequently, the picture of respiratory failure in SMA is usually one of a child who manages to get by until he or she gets a cold. Unable to cough up the phlegm, the upper respiratory infection goes to pneumonia. Respiratory failure in SMA is usually an acute occurrence. Planning and predictability are often not a luxury.

If predictability is difficult, treatment is not. The problems encountered are mechanical, and treatment is also mechanical.

Since respiratory failure in neuromuscular disease is secondary to failure of the respiratory muscles, a mechanical ventilator is an excellent treatment modality, since it can easily replace these weakened muscles. Substitution of the mechanical ventilator for the respiratory muscles in these patients meets with easy success. The patient's weakness makes it virtually impossible to fight the machine, and the fatigued patient willingly accepts the rest. Another factor in the success is that the integrity of the lungs is usually preserved. Although the patient may have had several pneumonias, the lung parenchyma is young and usually still healthy. These patients suffer the irony of respiratory failure while still maintaining normal or close to normal lungs.

As in the other neuromuscular diseases, assisted mechanical ventilation can be accomplished in many different ways, including negative pressure and positive pressure systems. Of our 15 patients, negative pressure was used initially in only one patient. Two other patients began by using mouth positive pressure. All three of these patients eventually required tracheal positive pressure ventilation.

Tracheal positive ventilation is the most aggressive and invasive form of assisted ventilation. We feel that it is justified in this patient population as an initial form of ventilation because of some of the unique aspects of the muscle weakness seen in this disease. First, the severity of the chest wall collapse due both to the weakened intercostals and often the additional complication of scoliosis places severe demands on the ventilatory system chosen for the patient. More importantly, the lack of a functional cough often makes the need for clearance of secretions a more important initial need than the need for assistance in breathing. This fact was demonstrated clearly by the fact that six of our 15 patients actually required a tracheostomy prior to requiring a ventilator.

Three of our earlier cases presented with cardiac problems secondary to respiratory involvement. One presented in cardiopulmonary arrest, and two others in congestive heart failure. In all cases, the cardiac problem resolved once the patient was stable on assisted ventilation. Our more recent patients have not had cardiac problems.

The decision to begin a child on assisted ventilation was necessitated by acute respiratory failure in 10 of the 15 patients studied. Two patients required assisted ventilation after spinal fusion procedures. Three of our more recent cases were started on assisted mechanical ventilation as a planned early intervention.

Our first goal of educating the families was easily accomplished. Frequent discussions were held with the family about the prognosis of the disease and treatment options. Continual updating of their child's status was also done. Psychological counseling was offered, but none of our families opted for such sessions. A great variability in the number of sessions the families requested with the physician, however, did occur. Education also included contact with families of other patients already on assisted ventilation, if this was desired.

Accomplishing the goal of predicting respiratory failure was not easy, but in eight patients we were able to avoid a major decompensation in respiratory status by offering assisted ventilation early. At this time, we use a combination of two factors to alert us to the need to initiate assisted ventilation in SMA patients who desire medical intervention. The predictive factors that we use are the onset of hypoxia combined with the additional indication of a history of recurrent pneumonias. Our criteria for a definition of impending respiratory failure have become lenient. We now select a PO_2 of less than 70 mm Hg (or, albeit rarely, a PCO_2 greater than

50 mm Hg) as our standard for early respiratory failure. In this patient population, therefore, we define hypoxia as any PO_2 of less than 70 mm Hg. We do this because we know that in the neuromuscular patient the precipitating cause of respiratory failure is the weakness in the respiratory muscles. We also recognize that this weakness is not something that can be expected to improve. A PO_2 of 70 mm Hg taken at a time when the patient is in good health will not improve with time but can only be expected to worsen.

Combining our criteria in this way led us to offer the patient and the family in these last eight cases the option of early assisted ventilation. In these cases it did allow the patient to avoid an acute emergency situation.

Our SMA patients on assisted ventilation have done very well. Only two of the 15 have died. These two patients died after 5 and 14 years of assisted ventilation. Three of our patients required full-time ventilator assistance at the time of the initiation of assisted ventilation; the remaining 12 were able to be weaned to nighttime assistance and were able to remain on nighttime assistance only for an average of 8 years 7 months. Nine patients continue to be on nighttime ventilation only, with three patients having used nighttime assistance for 20 years.

There are many debates that stimulate discussion among followers of neuromuscular patients. One debate concerns whether resting weakened muscles might speed loss of function. In SMA in particular, there is a second debate that centers on whether SMA is a static or progressive disease. If we look at these issues solely as they pertain to the respiratory muscles and look at the data on nighttime assisted ventilation, we can say that resting the respiratory muscles overnight has not sped the decline in function. In fact, in four patients, we were able to find forced vital capacity data that both preceded and followed the initiation of assisted ventilation. The forced vital capacities in these patients were obtained during the day while the patient was off all equipment. In all four cases, the data showed an increase in forced vital capacity after the initiation of assisted ventilation. The increase was maintained for as long as five years. This data, plus the information that the patients remained nighttime assisted only for so long a period of time, indicate that the short period of rest afforded by a night without the struggle to breath has not sped the progression of respiratory muscle weakness, but appears to have offered renewal and increased ability the morning after.

As far as the controversy concerning whether SMA is a static or progressive disease, the current popular view has become a compromise position that SMA is a disease of many plateaus in muscle strength. These plateaus, which may last several decades, are interspersed with periods of decline in function. Our data seems to concur with this concept. Our data shows a progression of respiratory muscle weakness that then plateaus during a time period where only nighttime assisted ventilation is required in the majority of our patients. Further decline eventually occurs, with a need for increasing time on the ventilator. The plateau period before fulltime ventilation became necessary has lasted several decades in several patients.

As for quality of life, it is necessary to see what life on a ventilator offers these patients. All but two of our patients remained at home after the initiation of assisted ventilation. One remained in our rehabilitation hospital. The second patient had been in a foster home prior to the initiation of assisted ventilation. He returned to that foster home for several years before being placed in a nursing home. Four of our older patients no longer live at home but are living independently on their own.

All but one of our patients attended regular school. The patient who attended a special school for orthopedically handicapped children remained at our hospital and attended school on the hospital grounds. Of the 10 patients older than 18, three graduated from college, two are presently in college, three graduated from high school, and two dropped out of school after completing the eleventh grade.

One patient is married and has one natural child and has adopted a second child. One patient is employed at a college as a vocational counselor. Two patients were involved in volunteer work, one with Planned Parenthood, and the second still is working as a volunteer psychologist at his church.

Our retrospective chart review revealed our patients to be active participants in life. Quality of life issues are at best a matter of judgment. We feel that our patients have goals similar to the nondisabled population, including education, independence, and social interaction. They have shown they have the ability to achieve these goals.

NOTES

1. Bach, J.R., J. O'Brien, R. Krotenberg, and A.S. Alba, "Management of End Stage Respiratory Failure in Duchenne Muscular Dystrophy," *Muscle Nerve* 1987;10:177–82.

2. Curran, F.J., "Night Ventilation by Body Respirators for Patients in Chronic Respiratory Failure Due to Late Stage Duchenne Muscular Dystrophy," *Arch Phys Med Rehabil* 1981;62:270–4.

3. Bach, J., A. Alba, L.A. Pilkington, and M. Lee, "Long-term Rehabilitation in Advanced Stage of Childhood Onset, Rapidly Progressive Muscular Dystrophy," *Arch Phys Med Rehabil* 1981;62:328–31.

4. Kerby, G.R., L.S. Mayer, and S.K. Pingleton, "Nocturnal Positive Pressure Ventilation via Nasal Mask," *AM Rev Respir Dis* 1987;135:738–40.

5. Iannaccone, S.T., and T. Guilfoile, "Long-term Mechanical Ventilation in Infants with Neuromuscular Disease," *J Child Neurol* 1988;3:30–2.

6. Gilgoff, I.S., E. Kahlstrom, E. MacLaughlin, and T.G. Keens, "Long-term Ventilatory Support in Spinal Muscular Atrophy," *J of Peds* 1989; 115:904–909.

7. Gilgoff, I., W. Prentice, and A. Beydur, "Patient and Family Participation in the Management of Respiratory Failure in Duchenne's Muscular Dystrophy," *Chest* 1989;95:519–24.

8. DeTroyer, A., and A. Heilporn, "Respiratory Mechanics in Quadriplegia: the Respiratory Function of the Intercostal Muscles," *Am Rev Respir Dis* 1980;122:591–600.

9. Siebens, A., N.A. Kirby, and D.A. Poulos, "Cough Following Transection of Spinal Cord at C-6," *Arch Phys Med Rehabil* 1964;45:1–8.

14

PSYCHOSOCIAL STRESSES AND COPING RESOURCES IN FAMILIES CARING FOR VENTILATOR-ASSISTED CHILDREN AT HOME

Susan E. Keens, M.A.
Mary T. Jansen, L.V.N.
Lee E. Lipsker, Ph.D.
Eric M. Levander
Jon E. Woo, A.B.
Frank T. Hsieh, B.A.
Irene S. Gilgoff, M.D.
Thomas G. Keens, M.D.

INTRODUCTION

Home care of ventilator-assisted children alters family lifestyles and may place severe stress on caregivers, yet this population has not been studied extensively (1,2,3). Advances in medical technology permit ventilator-assisted children to be cared for at home (4,5,6,7); however, the impact of such care on family lifestyle, the stresses caused by home care, marriage, and the ability of the care providers to cope is not known (1,2). However, it is known that many such caregivers do appear to experience a high degree of stress (8,9,10).

PERCEIVED SOURCES OF STRESS

We performed a preliminary survey of 28 primary caregivers of ventilator-assisted children at home to determine their perceived sources of stress related to such care (8,9,10). A number of perceived stressors were identified.

Home care of ventilator-assisted children alters traditional roles of parents and health care professionals. Many parents identified stressors associated with these alterations in health care provider roles. For example, adequate local emergency care was not available for about half of the ventilator-assisted children (8). The time required for clinic visits and to provide home treatments stressed one-half to two-thirds of the caregivers. Approximately three-quarters of the families were stressed by fear of equipment failure (8). Excessively long emergency response time from respiratory equipment vendors for ventilator malfunction stressed most caregivers. Nearly all ventilator-assisted children receiving in-home nursing assistance complained of a lack of privacy. The inability of nursing agencies to staff shifts with competent nurses stressed many caregivers (8). Further, some families found nurses who had fallen asleep on the job. Thus, many caregivers of ventilator-assisted children at home appear to experience stresses from their perceptions of unmet demands from health care providers (8).

The effect that home care for ventilator-assisted children has on family lifestyle is not known. Most parents were unable to pursue career choices, education, or job changes because of care requirements for their ventilator-assisted children (9). Over one-half of the parents were unable to change employers because the medical insurance of the new employer would not cover the ventilator-assisted children's preexisting condition (9). After the ventilator-assisted child first came home, it took an average of over four months before parents went out and left the ventilator-assisted child in another person's care (9). Of the ventilator-assisted children with in-home nursing assistance, funding agency restrictions prevented all from going on overnight trips or vacations with their families. Most families reported that the siblings felt ignored, and, in many families, siblings had behavior problems. Over one-half of the parents canceled special events and day-to-day activities for siblings because their ventilator-assisted child was sick. Thus, home care of ventilator-assisted children is associated with major alterations in family lifestyle (9) that affect all family members and interfere not only with day-to-day activities, but also with major factors, such as parents' careers (9).

It is not known if the stresses affect divorce, separation, or marital discord. Some families appear to cope with the stresses better than others. One-half of the parents received the most psychosocial support from their spouse, and nearly all rated their spouse as very supportive (10). Other important sources of psychosocial support included hospital nurses and physicians, home care nurses, and relatives (10). Most parents had support resources they could call at anytime. Approximately one-half of the parents had someone who could care for their ventilator-assisted children in emergencies, and they also had someone they could call to provide respite (10). Of the ventilator-assisted children receiving home shift nursing, nearly all complained of lack of privacy (10).

For the majority of parents, having their ventilator-assisted child at home was less stressful than separation from the children when they they were in the hospital (10). Nearly all of the parents believed that they provided better medical care for their ventilator-assisted children at home than they received in the hospital (8). The majority of the parents felt that having their ventilator-assisted children at home was generally a positive experience (9).

The true incidence of stress symptoms and coping resources to combat stress in caregivers of ventilator-assisted children at home is unknown. It is not known if these stresses affect divorce, separation, or marital discord, and how the families cope with them. In order to answer these questions, we surveyed primary caregivers of 53 ventilator-assisted children at home to assess psychosocial stresses and coping resources (11,12,13).

HYPOTHESES

In families caring for ventilator-assisted children at home, we hypothesized that:

1. Most caregivers would experience a high degree of distress (11).
2. The degree of caregiver distress would be related to the ventilator-assisted child's diagnosis (11).
3. Caregiver distress would be related to the length of time the ventilator-assisted child was at home (11).
4. Families would suffer a high incidence of divorce, separation, and marital discord (13).
5. Caregivers with a low degree of distress could cope better than caregivers with a high degree of distress (12).
6. Caregivers who had a high degree of marital discord would also suffer a high degree of distress (13).

METHODS

We used standardized, self-report questionnaires in the survey (11,12,13). The following measures were taken.

1. A questionnaire asking about primary caretakers' perceived sources of stress related to providing care for their ventilator-assisted child at home

was designed by the investigators (8,9,10). This is not a standardized or validated measure.

2. Symptom Checklist 90-R is a multi-dimensional self-report symptom inventory, designed to measure symptomatic psychological distress (14).

3. Coping Resources Inventory investigates coping resources in a population (15).

4. Family Environment Scale, Form R, assesses the social environmental characteristics of all types of families (16).

5. Locke-Wallace Inventory describes the degree of marital satisfaction or discord across 14 categories of common marital concern (17).

6. Social Support Questionnaire assesses the perceived number of social supports and satisfaction with social support that is available to the respondent (18).

7. Multi-Dimensional Health Locus of Control Scales assesses the locus of control related to health, along three dimensions (19).

STUDY GROUP

Data were compiled from 35 caregivers who responded (11,12,13). The age range of the ventilator-assisted children at the time of the study was 1-24 years. There were more males than females. The children had been home on assisted ventilation for an average of a little over four years. The majority of parents reported that their children were medically stable for the two months prior to completing the questionnaires.

Approximately one-third of the children required mechanical assisted ventilation for central hypoventilation syndrome; about one-half had ventilatory muscle weakness; the remainder had chronic lung disease. Approximately one-third of the children required continuous, 24-hour-per-day assisted ventilation; the remainder required assisted ventilation only while they slept. The majority of the ventilator-assisted children used portable positive pressure ventilators via tracheostomy (4,5,7); a few used negative pressure chest shell or pulmo-wrap ventilators (20); one used diaphragm pacing (21).

CAREGIVER DISTRESS

Caregivers were defined as having a high degree of distress if they had SCL-9OR scores greater than 60 (11,14). Over one-third of the caregivers had SCL-9OR scores greater than 60, indicating both an increased number of symptoms and intensity of distress (14). Thus, while a number of the caregivers did exhibit high distress, most did not (11).

Caregiver distress was not related to the age of the ventilator-assisted child (11). Similarly, it was not related to the child's diagnosis, and the intensity of caregiver distress decreased as the length of time the ventilator-assisted child was at home increased (11).

Caregivers experiencing low distress had significantly higher coping resources than those experiencing high distress (11,14,15). Marital discord, indicated by low Locke-Wallace Inventory scores, was not significantly different between families with high or low caregiver distress (11,14,17). Similarly, the number of social supports and caregiver satisfaction with such support (as indicated by the Social Support Questionnaire) were no different between families with high or low caregiver distress (11,14,18). Caregiver locus of control related to health was not related to caregiver distress (11,14,19). Thus, marital discord, social support, and health locus of control were not related to caregiver distress (11).

COPING RESOURCES

Using the Coping Resources Inventory, over one-quarter of the caregivers had low coping resources, indicated by CRI total scores less than 161 (12,15). Stress was significantly increased in caregivers with low coping resources (12,14,15). Thus, caregivers with low distress had higher coping resources than caregivers with high distress (12).

Caregivers with low coping resources had higher marital discord (12,15,17) and received less support from their families (12,15,16) than caregivers with high coping resources. There were no significant differences in number of social supports (12,15,18), satisfaction with social support (12,15,18), or family conflict (12,15,16) between caregivers with low versus high coping resources. Thus, caregivers with low coping resources had more marital discord and less family cohesion, but no difference in social support (12).

MARITAL DISCORD AND DIVORCE

There were only a few divorces and marital separations in these families caring for ventilator-assisted children at home, which is less than might be expect in a population caring for children with serious chronic diseases (13). However, there was a high incidence of marital discord (13,17), defined by a primary caregiver Locke Wallace Inventory score less than 115 (17).

Distress was higher and stress symptoms more intense in caregivers from families with marital discord than in those without (13,14,17). Coping resources were also lower, and the caregivers were less likely to be guided by stable and consistent values derived from religious or cultural traditions than caregivers from families without marital discord (13,15,17).

Family cohesion was slightly lower in caregivers with marital discord than in caregivers without marital discord, but family conflict was not different (13,16,17). There were no differences in number of social supports or satisfaction with social support (13,17,18). Thus, for caregivers of ventilator-assisted children at home, marital discord was related to decreased family cohesion, but not to family conflict or social support (13), nor was it related to the age, length of time at home, or diagnosis of the ventilator-assisted child (13).

CONCLUSIONS

1. In the population of caregivers under study, a number experienced high distress, but most did not (11).
2. Caregiver distress was not related to the ventilator-assisted child's diagnosis (11).
3. Caregiver distress decreased as the length of time the ventilator-assisted child was at home increased (11).
4. Many of the caregivers had low coping resources. In these caregivers, distress was inversely related to coping resources (12).
5. In the population, there were only a few divorces and marital separations. However, there was a high incidence of marital discord (13).
6. Caregivers with low coping resources had more distress, higher marital discord, and less family cohesion than those with high coping resources (12).

SPECULATION

We speculate that improving coping resources may reduce stress in caregivers caring for ventilator-assisted children at home. Reducing marital discord and improving family support may improve coping resources (11,12,13). Further, as ventilator-assisted children are at home longer, caregivers experience less stress because they have more time to develop coping strategies (11).

ACKNOWLEDGMENTS

The authors thank Drs. Sally L. Davidson Ward, C. Michael Bowman, Cheryl D. Lew, and Arnold C.G. Platzker, for providing medical care for many of the patients described in this study; Pamela K. DeWitt, R.N. and M.N., for her nursing expertise in the care of these children; and Richard A. Hunt, Ph.D., and David W. Foy, Ph.D., for their advice and support.

This study was funded, in part, by the Respiratory Control Disorders Fund, of the Division of Neonatology and Pediatric Pulmonology, Childrens Hospital Los Angeles.

Results of this study were presented, in part, at the 1989 and 1990 Annual Meetings of the Western Society for Pediatric Research, Carmel, California,

February 7, 1989, and February 6, 1990, and at the 1989 Annual Meeting of the American Thoracic Society, Cincinnati, Ohio, May 15, 1989.

NOTES

1. U.S. Department of Health and Human Services, *Report of the Task Force on Technology Dependent Children: Fostering Home and Community-based Care for Technology Dependent Children,* Health Care Financing Administration Publication No. 88-02171, 1988.

2. Aday, L.A., and D.H. Wegener, "Home care for Ventilator-assisted Children: Implications for the Children, Their Families, and Health Policy," *Children's Health Care,* 1988, 17: 112–120.

3. Jansen, M.T., P.K DeWitt, R.J. Meshul, J.B. Krasnoff, A.M. Lau, and T.G. Keens, "Meeting Psychosocial and Developmental Needs of Children during Prolonged Intensive Care Unit Hospitalization," *Children's Health Care,* 1989,18: 91–95.

4. Davidson Ward, S.L., and T.G. Keens, "Ventilatory Management at Home," in R.A. Ballard, ed., *Pediatric Care of the ICN Graduate* (Philadelphia: W.B. Saunders, 1988), pp. 166–176.

5. O'Donohue, W.J., Jr., R.M. Giovannoni, A. I. Goldberg, T.G. Keens, B.I. Make, A.L. Plummer, and W.S. Prentice, "Long-term Mechanical Ventilation: Guidelines for Management in the Home and at Alternate Community Sites," *Chest,* 90 (Suppl), 1986, 1S-37S.

6. Plummer, A.L., W.J. O'Donohue, Jr., and T.L. Petty, "Conference Report: Consensus Conference on Problems in Home Mechanical Ventilation," *Am. Rev. Respirat. Dis.,* 1989, 140: 555–560.

7. Gilgoff, I.S., E. Kahlstrom, E. MacLaughlin, and T.G. Keens, "Long-term Ventilatory Support in Spinal Muscular Atrophy," *J. Pediatr.,* 1989, 115: 904–909.

8. Keens, S.E., M.T. Jansen, L.E. Lipsker, and T.G. Keens, "Parental Stresses from Providing Home Care to Ventilator Dependent Children," *Am. Rev. Respirat. Dis.,* 1989, 139(4): 543A.

9. Keens, S.E., M.T. Jansen, L.E. Lipsker, I.S. Gilgoff, and T.G. Keens, "Lifestyle Alterations in Families With Ventilator Dependent Children at Home," *Am. Rev. Respirat. Dis.,* 1989, 139(4): 195A.

10. Keens, S.E., M.T. Jansen, L.E. Lipsker, and T.G. Keens, "Marital Stability and Psychosocial Support for Parents of Ventilator Dependent Children at Home," *Am. Rev. Respirat. Dis.*, 1989, 139(4): 543A.

11. Keens, S.E., M.T. Jansen, L.E. Lipsker, I.S. Gilgoff, and T.G. Keens, "Comparison of Stressed and Nonstressed Parents Caring for Ventilator Assisted Children at Home," *Pediatr. Res*, 1990, 27(4): 11A.

12. Keens, S.E., M.T. Jansen, L.E. Lipsker, and T.G. Keens, "Coping Resources to Combat Stress in Parents Caring for Ventilator Assisted Children at Home," *Pediatr. Res.*, 1990, 27(4): 11A.

13. Keens, S.E., M.T. Jansen, L.E. Lipsker, and T.G. Keens, "Marital Discord and Increased Stress in Parents of Ventilator Assisted Children at Home," *Pediatr. Res.*, 1990, 27(4): 11A.

14. Derogatis, L.R., and P.N. Cleary, *SCL-90 (Revised) Manual-I.*(Baltimore: Johns Hopkins University Press, 1977).

15. Hammer, A.L, and M.S. Marting, *Manual for the Coping Resources Inventory* (Palo Alto: Consulting Psychologists Press, 1988).

16. Moos, R.H., and B.S. Moos, *Family Environment Scale Manual*, Second Edition (Palo Alto: Consulting Psychologists Press, 1986).

17. Locke, J.J., and K.M. Wallace, "Short-term Marital Adjustment and Prediction Tests: Their Reliability and Validity," *J. Marriage and Family Living*, 1959, 21: 251–256.

18. Sarason, I.G., H.M. Levine, R.B. Basham, and B.R. Sarason, "Assessing Social Support: The Social Support Questionnaire," *J. Personal Soc. Psychol.*, 1983, 44: 127–139.

19. Wallston, K.A., B.S. Walston, and R. DeVellis, "Development of the MHLC Scales," *Health Education Monographs*, 1978, 6: 160–170.

20. Splaingard, M.L, R.C. Frates, Jr., L.S. Jefferson, C.L. Rosen, and G.M. Harrison, "Home Negative Pressure Ventilation: Report of 20 years of Experience in Patients with Neuromuscular Disease," *Arch Phys. Med. Rehabil.*, 1985, 66: 239–242.

21. Glenn, W.W.L., and M.L. Phelps, "Diaphragm Pacing by Electrical Stimulation of the Phrenic Nerve," *Neurosurgery* 17: 974–984, 1985.

15

ETHICAL PROBLEMS CONCERNING TREATMENT OF AND ATTITUDE TOWARD CHRONIC RESPIRATORY INSUFFICIENCY IN MUSCULAR DYSTROPHY

Bente Madsen

My respiratory problems began in March 1974 with a common cold. Due to my poor ability to cough, I developed pneumonia within a few days. I was put into intensive care, naso-tracheally intubated, and ventilated. Shortly after dismissal, I developed symptoms of hypoventilation.

During the following 18 months, I was nasally intubated and artificially ventilated five times. Following each period of treatment, the symptoms recurred sooner than the last time and were more severe. The final six months before I had a tracheostomy, I was almost permanently hospitalized, and I remember nothing but one long, continuous, thanatofobic nightmare.

I was never informed about the cause of the symptoms, my prognosis, or optional treatment modalities. When tracheostomy was performed, I was so sick that I was unable to relate to my own situation in any meaningful way, and thus the decision to tracheostomize was exclusively medical.

After the tracheostomy, I got well. My body and brain resumed functioning, and I experienced an intense anger that I had not had the tracheostomy earlier, instead of suffering anguish for six months. My questions about why my family and I had not been told about the possibility of permanent artificial ventilation were answered by the head of the medical department, with the explanation that the doctors had had grave doubts. They had discussed whether it would be medically justifiable to prolong the life of someone who was impaired by a severe physical handicap. They felt they could not discuss their doubt with me. Mere fortuity therefore decided that I should be alive today.

Because of these personal experiences, I have for the last ten years taken a keen interest in the treatment of and the attitude toward people suffering from a chronic respiratory handicap.

In the last few years, more openness has evolved concerning the counseling of the respiratory handicapped and their families. It has been my experience, however, that a number of myths and prejudices continue to prevail concerning permanent ventilator therapy. Furthermore, it is my experience that new users often seem to lack information about their respiratory aids and the course and prognosis of their illness. Thus they run the risk of being victims of their doctors' attitudes toward quality of life.

In Denmark, positive pressure ventilation with a tracheostomy is the most common treatment of chronic respiratory insufficiency. Only in a very few instances is negative pressure ventilation with a pulmo-wrap employed, as this later method restricts the user to a supine position. Greater frankness about respiratory illness has resulted in an increasing number of people being treated before the problems occur in their acute form, and some people may live for several years with positive pressure ventilation and a nasal mask during the night and periods of rest.

To a great extent, it is the doctor who decides when, and to whom, ventilator therapy should be offered. Clear guidelines are lacking, and a number of people with respiratory problems are never informed about the possibility of ventilator treatment.

For several years I have worked as an advisor in the respiratory field for the Danish Association of Muscular Dystrophy, a group of respiratorily handicapped people whom I will discuss in the following material.

Treatment of respiratory insufficiency in muscular dystrophy is centralized in two of the largest hospitals in Denmark. Due to an accounting system that requires the counties to pay for therapy at the central departments, a few people are treated locally. They run the risk of receiving poor or no advice or treatment.

Myths and prejudices surround the use of permanent artificial ventilation. The earliest of these stems from the polio epidemic in the 1950s, when the respiratorily handicapped lay in large iron lungs in hospital wards. The later myths arise from the news media, with sensation-seeking reports of sudden accidents, paralysis, and misery, with ensuing dependence on doctors and high technology equipment.

In my capacity as an advisor, I have visited users of ventilation equipment who have different types of muscular dystrophy and live at home or in hospitals. Prior to my visit, they had all had a consultation with a doctor concerning tracheostomy and the use of permanent ventilation. Some had a better understanding of their situation than others, but in general they were surprised that I was mobile and able to talk. The doctors claim that they explain and advise adequately, but the fact remains that the users do not understand the explanations and are left with mental images of further dependency and isolation.

Users and doctors alike are influenced by such images. It is difficult to give and receive information in an objective manner. Anxious conceptions may also be the reason doctor and user often postpone the decision to employ ventilation equipment until the user suffers severe symptoms of hypoventilation and is in no condition to relate meaningfully to a new situation.

A sufferer of muscular dystrophy who has a tracheostomy soon becomes dependent on the ventilator, which may explain the reluctance on the doctor's part to use such measures. From a medical point of view, therapy should traditionally result in progress. Some doctors find it difficult to envisage how increased dependency on a ventilator can be progress—even though the user has evidently improved.

In 1989, the Danish Association of Muscular Dystrophy made a survey—"Existence for Permanent Ventilator-Users—The Users' Point of View"—among the 16 permanent ventilator users suffering from muscular dystrophy in Denmark. (Of these, 11 have had a tracheostomy, one-quarter of them without any preparation.)

More than one-half of the 16 felt they had been in need of respiratory aid 6 to 12 months prior to receiving it. The study demonstrated that no one regretted having become a permanent ventilator user. Two-thirds of the users explained that they had more energy and zest for life. They were almost never hospitalized anymore, and fear of death and the feeling of suffocation had disappeared. It had also become easier to plan for the future and make demands on each other, since death had been postponed. They all agreed that only advantages arose from artificial ventilation. Everyone in the survey took an active part in organizational work, education, job, or family life, and all had plans for the future.

A few now and then did experience limitations in mobility due to extra equipment such as a suction unit, batteries, the proximity to power current and plug, and the fact that they were literally tied to their aid.

Considerations about age and diagnosis had decided that I was "suitable" for permanent ventilation. I was among the first with muscular dystrophy to have a tracheostomy, and although greater openness evolved in the ensuing years, those who have been helped are mainly people with a slowly progressing disease.

Until a few years ago, young people with Duchenne's muscular dystrophy were deemed "unsuitable" for artificial ventilation, due to the aggressive nature of that disease.

When a person with a respiratory handicap is tracheostomized, it is easy to get stuck in the "patient role." When the user is discharged from the hospital, the doctor takes responsibility for the respiratory treatment, since it is his or her ethical and legal duty, as imposed by the Ministry of the

Interior. This entails regular visits to the outpatient clinic, not because the user feels sick or in need of medical attention, but so that the blood gasses can be measured, the tracheal tube changed, and the ventilator checked to see that it gives out the proper amount of air.

Some users are told that they or their helpers are not allowed to regulate or repair the ventilator. Others have no idea how to perform these adjustments, should the need arise. In some instances, the hospital demands that a trained nurse visit the user every day, in order to clean the tracheostomy and change the stomal serviette.

Although there are only two central departments that deal with the treatment of chronic respiratory insufficiency, there may be differences as to how the ventilators are applied to users with a tracheostomy. In some cases, all the tubes to the pressure control system are kept. This looks bulky and dramatic and makes the user feel like someone in an intensive care ward. The use of silver tracheal cannulas has been abandoned, and plastic tubes that often look huge are employed.

In many instances, the air hoses are inappropriately thick, even though made of a soft and pliable material. In other cases, a solution has been found—removing the pressure tubes and expiration valve. Expiration then takes place through fauces and nose.

It must be presumed that all treatment is undertaken with the best medical intentions; thus, innovative thinking is imperative to help remove the doctor's personal attitude toward quality of life from his counseling.

We must learn and teach that the use of permanent ventilation, with or without tracheostomy, has nothing to do with sickness or isolation. The ventilator is an aid compensating for weak muscular power, in analogy to the wheelchair.

The predictability of the course muscular dystrophy will take in many cases affords the doctor time to advise both the user and the relatives about the prognosis of the disease and the possibility of using artificial ventilation when the need arises.

A lot has been said about how to determine when the need for artificial ventilation is real. From the user's point of view, it is traumatic to experience the symptoms of hypoventilation, and it is therefore unacceptable to wait until blood-gas values and vital capacity have sunk beneath a given level.

The"suitable" ventilator user is not necessarily the youngest, the most active, or the one with the slowest progress of the disease. Rather, it is a question of whether the patient has the energy and desire to go on living with a severe physical handicap. This is a decision that can only be made by the user while it is still possible to take a stand about one's condition. Varying random ideas about quality of life and concern about government economy are ethically and medically unjustifiable.

When a user has made the decision about permanent ventilator use, based on a thorough understanding of his or her disease and prognosis, the transition from night ventilation with nasal mask or pulmo-wrap to tracheostomy will be facilitated. Likewise, the well-informed user who does not wish to prolong life should be able to say "thank you, no" to the offer of permanent ventilator use and be helped to a death with dignity and without anxiety.

Regardless of the method of ventilation used, it is important to ensure that the user has the ability to get around. Negative pressure ventilation is thus suited for those who can do with artificial ventilation at night and during rest.

Breathing is a basic function, and it is important not to feel estranged from the ventilator that is now part of you. New users should be thoroughly educated in how the machine functions and must possess the necessary equipment. Insecurity may lead to isolation and bitterness, which is not the goal of a life-prolonging procedure such as permanent ventilation.

When a person suffers from muscular dystrophy and artificial ventilation becomes necessary, he or she is already totally dependent on others, so permanent ventilator use has no real significance concerning dependence on others and does not limit the possibilities of spontaneity and leading an extroverted, active life. However, the user must have optimal mobility and feel secure.

It is unworthy to be forced to live as an "eternal patient" due to others' concepts of safety and responsibility. The role of patient is not attractive, and no one wants to be placed in it any longer than strictly necessary. Instead, therapists must learn to help users become their own experts.

Tracheostomized, well-educated, secure ventilator users are their own best gasometer, seeking medical help only when necessary, and able to train their helpers themselves. A nursing education is not required to become a helper to a tracheostomized ventilator user, but motivation and logical thinking are essential. Tracheostomized users with none, or a very limited amount of, spontaneous respiration may benefit from the ventilator control system. But users with some spontaneous respiration or those who wish to have the alarm shut off must be able to have the pressure control tubes disconnected. Pressure tubes, overly large air hoses, large expiration valves, and plastic tracheal tubes often seem very dramatic.

Doctors often forget cosmetic considerations and fail to advise users of different types of air hoses, connections, and tubes. It is important for the handicapped to look attractive, but it may be difficult to retain self-respect if the aid the person must use becomes the dominant factor. It is therefore important to find the most appropriate solution for each user.

Greater frankness concerning the respiratory area has led to more people being offered permanent respiratory aid. But there are almost as many opinions about "suitability," need, methods, and aids as there are therapists.

Since the polio epidemic of the 1950s, statistics have demonstrated that permanent ventilator users lead lives as active and extroverted as other physically handicapped people. It seems strange, therefore, that neither experience nor debate has been able to ensure users a high standard of advice and treatment, allowing them to make the vital decisions for themselves.

16

CHRONIC VENTILATORY SUPPORT AT HOME FOR INFANTS AND CHILDREN WITH VENTILATORY MUSCLE WEAKNESS

Thomas G. Keens, M.D.
Mary T. Jansen, L.V.N.
Jon E. Woo, A.B.
Sally L. Davidson Ward, M.D.
Pamela K. Dewitt, R.N., M.N.
Irene S. Gilgoff, M.D.

Immaturity of the lungs and ventilatory muscles in infants and young children may make the institution of home ventilation difficult, or at least require alteration in ventilator techniques. We have ventilated 28 infants and children with ventilatory muscle weakness at home. Assisted ventilation was begun at a mean age of 7.0±1.5 [SE] years. In 13 infants (46 percent), assisted ventilation was initiated at less than two years of age. In 19 children (68 percent), assisted ventilation was begun *nonelectively* because of the inability to wean the child from a ventilator after an episode of acute respiratory failure. In nine children (32 percent), assisted ventilation was begun *electively* to improve the quality of life and preserve physiologic function. Nearly all of the children were ventilated at home, using electronic portable positive pressure ventilators via tracheostomy. Because there is a large, variable leak around uncuffed tracheostomy tubes used in infants and small children, a time cycled, pressure limited mode of ventilation was used by modifying ventilator settings. This allowed adequate ventilation of all children without the use of cuffed tracheostomy tubes, continuous gas flow, or PEEP, preserving the advantage of portability in electronic home ventilators. After 2.4±0.3 years of assisted ventilation at home, four children (14 percent) died and three children (11 percent) were able to be weaned from assisted ventilation. Twenty-two children over three years of age (96 percent) attend school or have graduated from high school. Hospital admissions for the children on home ventilators were infrequent. We conclude that chronic ventilatory support can be safely instituted at home for children with ventilatory muscle weakness, and that these children can attend school, have fewer hospitalizations, and achieve a high quality of life.

INTRODUCTION

The physiologic consequences of ventilatory muscle weakness in infants and children include: decreased ability to expand their lungs, resulting in atelectasis; decreased cough, resulting in retained pulmonary secretions and increased pulmonary infections; and inadequate ventilation, especially during sleep (1,2,3). Mechanical-assisted ventilation can reverse these consequences, though not cure the disorder. Many centers have considerable experience with home ventilation of adolescents and young adults with neuromuscular diseases (4,5,6). However, immaturity of the lungs and ventilatory muscles in infants and young children may make the institution of home ventilation difficult, or at least require alteration in ventilator techniques (1,7,8). Childrens Hospital Los Angeles and Rancho Los Amigos Medical Center have ventilated a large number of infants and young children with ventilatory muscle weakness at home (4).

STUDY AIMS

We reviewed our clinical experience with 28 infants and children with ventilatory muscle weakness managed with chronic ventilatory support at home in order to answer the following questions:

1. Can mechanical-assisted ventilation be achieved safely in the home?
2. What ventilation techniques result in successful home care?
3. Can hospitalizations be reduced by using mechanical-assisted ventilation at home?
4. Can mechanically assisted children participate in normal activities at home?

STUDY GROUP

Twenty-eight infants and children with ventilatory muscle weakness were managed with mechanical-assisted ventilation in the home. Sixty-four percent were males. Assisted ventilation was begun at a mean age of 7.0±1.5

[SE] years, and they first went home at 7.3±1.4 years of age. In 13 infants (46 percent), mechanical-assisted ventilation was begun before two years of age; and ten infants (36 percent) first went home on assisted ventilation at less than two years of age.

The children had the following diagnoses. Nine children had spinal muscular atrophy; five had muscular dystrophy; five had high spinal cord injury from multiple causes; three had nemaline rod myopathy; and eight had other myopathies.

INITIATION OF CHRONIC VENTILATORY SUPPORT

In 19 children (68 percent), mechanical-assisted ventilation was begun *nonelectively,* because of the inability to wean the child from a ventilator after an episode of acute respiratory failure. Acute respiratory failure was caused by pneumonia in eight children, birth injury in four children, following surgical procedures or trauma in four children, and associated with progressive cor pulmonale in three children.

In contrast, mechanical-assisted ventilation was begun *electively* in nine children (32 percent) to preserve physiologic function and improve their quality of life (5). In six of these children, assisted ventilation was begun because of decreased daytime activity or intermittent respiratory distress at night, and in three children to prevent frequent severe pneumonias. Elective institution of mechanical-assisted ventilation was discussed with the patient and family before the need arose, thus providing the opportunity to begin assisted ventilation early, before significant complications of hypoventilation occurred (1,4).

MODALITIES OF CHRONIC VENTILATORY SUPPORT AT HOME

Three children were ventilated using a negative pressure pulmo-wrap ventilator (9). In one child, who used a negative pressure pulmo-wrap for one year, a tracheostomy and positive pressure ventilation were required because of the inability to maintain adequate gas exchange with negative pressure ventilation. In one infant with diaphragm paralysis, who required ventilation only during sleep, a negative pressure ventilator was fashioned from a pulmo-wrap ventilator. This resulted in successful ventilation during sleep and improved spontaneous ventilation during wakefulness. This infant was completely weaned from assisted ventilation after eight months of ventilatory support, and never required a tracheostomy.

Twenty-five children (89 percent) used electronic portable positive pressure ventilators via tracheostomy (1,10). However, infants and young children require different techniques of positive pressure ventilation to achieve adequate gas exchange and maintain ventilator portability. In infants and young children receiving positive pressure ventilation, uncuffed tracheostomies are used. Therefore, a portion of the ventilator-delivered breath escapes in the leak around the tracheostomy. Commercially available portable positive pressure ventilators for use at home are volume cycled. In some older children and adolescents, the leak around the tracheostomy is relatively constant and a high tidal volume setting can be used to compensate for the leak and achieve adequate ventilation. This tidal volume setting must be derived empirically, as there is no way to predict the portion of a ventilator-delivered breath that escapes through the leak. However, in infants and small children, the tracheostomy leak is quite variable, and since it is relatively large compared to the desired delivered tidal volume, it cannot be compensated for by a single tidal volume setting. The tracheostomy leak can be compensated for by using the ventilator in a pressure limited modality, also known as pressure plateau ventilation (1,10, 12).

Assuming relatively constant pulmonary mechanics, the lungs will be inflated to the same tidal volume on each breath if the same peak inspiratory pressure is used. Tidal volume is dictated by the patient's pressure-volume curve. Some portable positive pressure ventilators have a high pressure limit adjustment which is separate from the high pressure alarm. The pressure limit is adjusted down to the desired peak inspiratory pressure. A large tidal volume setting is then dialed in to compensate both for the leak and for lung inflation. The ventilator will now function in a *pressure plateau* mode. When the pressure limit is reached, the remainder of the ventilator tidal volume will be delivered to the room, rather than to the patient. If there is a large tracheostomy leak one moment, a large portion of the tidal volume will be delivered through the ventilator, but the lungs will be inflated to the desired pressure. If there is a small tracheostomy leak the next moment, a lesser portion of the tidal volume will be delivered, but the lungs will still be inflated to the desired pressure (1,10,12).

Using this technique, all 26 patients were able to be ventilated at home without cuffed tracheostomy tubes, continuous flow, or PEEP, thus preserving the advantage of portability in electronic home ventilators.

CLINICAL OUTCOME OF VENTILATOR-ASSISTED CHILDREN

Twenty-four of these children (86 percent), are currently in their natural parents' homes. Only three children required foster placement. One child, originally placed in her natural parents' home, is now in a state institution because of the inability of her family to provide care.

Children were managed at home with mechanical-assisted ventilation for a mean of 2.4±0.3 years. Eight children (29 percent) required full-time ventilation initially, and remain full-time ventilator dependent. Four children (14 percent) who required full-time ventilation initially have died. Nine children (32 percent) required part-time ventilation initially and remain part-time ventilator dependent. Four children (14 percent) began assisted ventilation part-time but progressed to become full-time ventilator dependent. Three children (11 percent) began assisted ventilation part-time but were able to be completely weaned from assisted ventilation.

Once at home on assisted ventilation, four children (14 percent) died. Death was due to cardiomyopathy from Duchenne's muscular dystrophy in two patients. One child died from sepsis. One child had a prolonged seizure associated with a high fever, and subsequently died. None died from a primary pulmonary problem or from malfunction of any home ventilator equipment.

Three children (11 percent) were able to be weaned from mechanical assisted ventilation at home. In all cases, weaning was associated with improvement in generalized skeletal muscle strength. Weaning occurred in one infant with nemaline myopathy at one year of age, one infant with diaphragm paralysis at two years of age, and one adolescent with an undiagnosed neuromuscular disease at 17 years of age.

Infants placed on assisted ventilation in the first few years of life spend relatively few days in the hospital in the early childhood years. At age eight to ten years, home ventilation was initiated in a group of children with nonprogressive neuromuscular disease. Rapid body growth increased the body mass that weakened muscles were required to move. An increase in mean hospital days was due to lengthy initial hospitalizations. Finally, at age 15-20, several adolescents with progressive neuromuscular disease began mechanical-assisted ventilation. Again, an increase in mean hospital days was due to lengthy initial hospitalizations.

When the length of time children spend in the hospital is calculated relative to the time assisted ventilation was begun, rather than age, one can see the effect of assisted ventilation on hospitalizations. The first year (when assisted ventilation was instituted) includes the relatively long initial hospitalization required to institute mechanical-assisted ventilation at home (11). Once home, children receiving mechanical-assisted ventilation spend relatively little time in hospitals, especially two or more years after the institution of chronic ventilatory support. This indicates that home care of children with ventilatory muscle weakness can be successfully achieved using mechanical-assisted ventilation.

QUALITY OF LIFE

For children, the measure of ability to participate in age appropriate activities is school attendance. Most of the children being described attended school. Six children (21 percent) were under three years of age, and thus too young to attend school. Of the remainder who were old enough to attend school or preschool, only one child was not in school. Three attend college, two others have graduated from high school, nine attend regular schools, and seven attend schools for the orthopedically handicapped. Thus, most children with ventilatory muscle weakness managed with home ventilation attend school, and most are in regular schools or college.

In addition to attending school, most of these children were able to participate in relatively normal childhood activities, such as active membership in the Brownies, going on carnival rides at amusement parks, going to Disneyland, decorating the power wheelchair with ventilator as an army tank for Halloween, and camping with the family. Many families have become extremely creative at ways to provide relatively normal activities for their ventilator-assisted children who remain at home.

CONCLUSIONS

Chronic ventilatory support can be safely instituted at home for children with ventilatory muscle weakness. Pressure plateau ventilation provides adequate gas exchange for these children without cuffed tracheostomy tubes, continuous flow, or PEEP. These children require relatively few hospitalizations once mechanical-assisted ventilation has been instituted at home. Children on home ventilators can attend regular schools or college, and achieve a high quality of life.

ACKNOWLEDGMENTS

The authors thank Drs. C. Michael Bowman, Cheryl D. Lew, and Arnold C.G. Platzker, for providing medical care for many of the patients described in this study.

This study was funded, in part, by the *Respiratory Control Disorders Fund*, of the Division of Neonatology and Pediatric Pulmonology, Childrens Hospital Los Angeles.

NOTES

1. Davidson Ward, S.L, and T.G. Keens, "Ventilatory Management at Home," in R.N. Ballard, ed., *Pediatric Care of the ICN Graduate* (Philadelphia: W.B. Saunders, 1988), pp. 166–176.

2. Roussos, C., and P.T. Macklem, "Inspiratory Muscle Fatigue," *The Handbook of Physiology: Section 3: The Respiratory System*, Volume III, Part 2 (Baltimore: American Physiological Society, 1986), pp. 511–528.

3. Phillipson, E.A., and G. Bowes, "Control of Breathing During Sleep," *The Handbook of Physiology: Section 3: The Respiratory System*, Volume II, Part 2 (Baltimore: American Physiological Society, 1986), pp. 649–690.

4. Gilgoff, I.S., E. Kahlstrom, E. MacLaughlin, and T.G. Keens, "Long-term Ventilatory Support in Spinal Muscular Atrophy," *J. Pediatr.*, 1989, 115: 904–909.

5. Gilgoff, I.S., W. Prentice, and A. Baydur, "Patient and Family Participation in the Management of Respiratory Failure in Duchenne's Muscular Dystrophy," *Chest*, 1989, 95: 519–524.

6. Harrison, B. D.W., J.V. Collins, K.G.E. Brown, and T.J.H. Clark, "Respiratory Failure in Neuromuscular Diseases," *Thorax*, 1971, 26: 579–584.

7. Keens, T.G., A.C. Bryan, H. Levison, and C.D. Ianuzzo, "Developmental Pattern of Muscle Fiber Types in Human Ventilatory Muscles," *J. Appl. Physiol.: Respirat. Environ. Exercise Physiol.*, 1978, 44: 909–913.

8. Scott, C.B., B.G. Nickerson, C.W. Sargent, A.C.G. Platzker, D. Warburton, and T.G. Keens, "Developmental Pattern of Maximal Transdiaphragmatic Pressure in Infants During Crying," *Pediatr. Res.*, 1983, 17: 707–709.

9. Splaingard, M.L., R.C. Frates, Jr., L.S. Jefferson, C.L. Rosen, and G.M. Harrison, "Home Negative Pressure Ventilation: Report of 20 Years of Experience in Patients With Neuromuscular Disease," *Arch Phys. Med. Rehabil.*, 1985, 66: 239–242.

10. O'Donohue, W.J., Jr., R.M. Giovannoni, A.I. Goldberg, T.G. Keens, B.I. Make, A.L. Plummer, and W.S. Prentice, "Long-term Mechanical Ventilation: Guidelines for Management in the Home and at Alternate Community Sites," *Chest*, 1986, 90 (Suppl.): 1S 37S.

11. DeWitt, P.K, M.T. Jansen, S.L. Davidson Ward, C.D. Lew, C.M. Bowman, A.C.G. Platzker, and T.G. Keens, "Obstacles to Discharge of Ventilator Dependent Children From the Hospital to Home," *Am. Rev. Respirat. Dis.*, 1989,139(4): 196A.

12. Gilgoff, I.S., R. Peng, T.G. Keens, "Hypoventilation and Apnea in Children during Mechanically Assisted Ventilation," *Chest*, 1992, 101:1500–1506.

17

DISCONTINUATION OF VENTILATORY SUPPORT

A Personal Perspective

Terry Kinzel, M.D., F.A.C.P., F.A.G.S.

INTRODUCTION

Medical ethicists are in general agreement that, ethically, there is no difference between the decision not to initiate a treatment and the withdrawal of a treatment once it has been started, especially if it has been determined that such a treatment is incapable of achieving the desired goal (1,2). This issue is common in the elderly with severe progressive disease and runs the gamut from decisions about physical therapy to that of resuscitation. However, the two areas most commonly discussed in decisions of this nature are artificial provision of food and water and ventilatory support in a person determined to be brain dead. Decisions involving food and water are complicated by nonmedical issues such as the concept of what is the most basic responsibility that one has to all persons. It is, however, in the discontinuation of previously initiated artificial ventilatory support that a deliberate decision, taken in a nonemergency setting, illustrates the most dramatic cause and effect in medicine.

I will use a personal experience during my internship 20 years ago to illustrate some of the issues involved.

REPORT OF A CASE

Mr. A was a 57-year-old white man who was brought to the hospital by paramedics in an ambulance after collapsing at home. Cardiopulmonary resuscitation had been rapidly initiated. In the emergency department he was intubated and successfully resuscitated, in that adequate cardiovascular function was re-established and maintained. However, he remained comatose, without any ventilatory effort, and was placed on a respirator. Subsequent evaluation revealed a subarrachnoid hemorrhage as the etiology of his arrest. Outside of moderate hypertension, he had previously had no significant illnesses.

The initial hospitalization was stormy, with wide swings in blood pressure and a high fever (presumably secondary to the subarrachnoid hemorrhage, as no infection was identified). He remained comatose and unresponsive, with no ventilatory effort. By the forth or fifth day, when recovery appeared unlikely, his family decided that further resuscitative efforts should not be undertaken if he suffered a cardiac arrest. At the time, this seemed fairly likely. However, over the next week, he stabilized, became afebrile and normotensive. All functions other than brain/respiratory, including liver and renal, were normal. At this point, approximately ten days following admission, death did not appear eminent, and the direction to take was discussed. A neurological consultation, including examination, caloric testing, and two flat-line EEGs separated by 24 hours while the patient was on no sedatives, concluded that the patient was brain dead, with no possibility of recovery.

At this point, the family decided that the ventilatory support should be withdrawn. After consultations with senior physicians, social services, and pastoral services, a written request from the family, including his wife, the next of kin, for withdrawal of the respirator was signed, witnessed, and entered into his chart.

As I had been the primary physician involved in the case, it did not seem appropriate for me to ask respiratory services to discontinue the respirator. Consequently, I disconnected the respirator and remained alone in the room for seven minutes until the heart of this brain-dead patient ceased functioning.

DISCUSSION

The issues in this case are clearer and more easily sorted out than in most. The patient was relatively young, had a sudden arrest, was attended to promptly, and prior to the arrest was in good health. This is the ideal situation to apply full resuscitative treatment, with a clear indication of the treatment needed and the time to institute it. This contrasts with the situation of someone with end stage chronic lung disease, who gradually becomes short of breath and whose PO_2 drops from a steady state of 50 mm Hg to 45 mm Hg. The indication and timing for the withdrawal of respiratory support also was clearer than usual. The cause of the arrest had been identified and was not reversible, and the patient met stringent criteria for brain death, but otherwise was physiologically stable (suggesting that death from a complication was not likely to occur in the near future). This also contrasts with the more common situation in which a person with end stage lung disease or multiple severe medical problems requires ventilatory support and becomes comatose. In these cases, the patient rarely meets the criteria for brain death, the precise cause for the coma is nearly impossible to identify, and irreversibility, while very likely, is not certain.

However, even in this ideal setting, the emotional impact upon me was great. I rarely experience it on a daily basis now, but writing this chapter brings it flooding back. As a geriatrician, I deal daily with dying patients. Few of their deaths have had the same impact on me as that of Mr. A. There have been numerous times that I have concurred with a patient's wish not to be placed on a respirator, at least some of whom may have had enough reversible illness to have had a chance to be taken off the respirator and lead a meaningful life, at least for a short time. In these instances, an ethicist would have encouraged me to initiate the respirator and, after a predetermined trial, discontinue it if predetermined goals were not achieved. Intellectually, this is sound reasoning. Emotionally, it will not wash. The deaths that resulted from the patients not being placed on a respirator should weigh more heavily on me than that of Mr. A. Yet they don't. In conversations with my colleagues I know that my experience is not unique; the emotional impact of removing a respirator is greater than that of not starting one. We are taught to first do no harm. No matter how clear the situation, it is not possible to be unaffected by an act that directly results in the cessation of physiological function.

While my intention is to describe a personal experience, the experience of the family also deserves acknowledgment. Despite the clear indications of irreversibility, the physicians involved and the hospital administration were uncomfortable with the potential liability. Thus, the formal means by which the family had to request withdrawal, including signed and witnessed written requests, was significant. While this process was technically correct, and perhaps unavoidable, it had the effect of increasing the burden on the family, impairing the ability of the staff to provide support during a terrifying time.

Ethically, there is no difference between withdrawing and foregoing to initiate a treatment for which the indication was not or is no longer present. Emotionally, there is. While in this case, emotion may not contribute to better medicine, as humans we are both intellectual and emotional beings. Those who would cast judgment must also practice.

NOTES

1. Fox, M., and H.L. Lipton, "The Decision to Perform Cardiopulmonary Resuscitation," *The New England Journal of Medicine* 1983, 309:607–608.

2. Purtilo, R.B., and C.K. Cassel, "Care for Incurably Ill Persons," in *Ethical Dimensions in the Health Professions* (Philadelphia: WB Saunders, 1981), pp. 92–109.

18

THE VENTILATOR—A WAY TO A POSITIVE LIFE

Jack Genskow

This chapter is somewhat informal in its presentation, because I want it to have a human rather than a professional technical quality. It deals directly with the question of placing someone with muscular dystrophy on a ventilator with a tracheostomy, but looks at the question from the viewpoint of a person who has used a ventilator and tracheostomy for 16 years. As you read this chapter, I ask that you put aside your professional roles and react as a human being sharing this process of life.

This chapter focuses on the experiences of Bente Madsen, a 40-year-old woman from Denmark who has muscular dystrophy. Many of her personal comments that follow are from an article in the 30th Anniversary Edition of the *Rehabilitation Gazette,* 1989, as well as from personal correspondence and subsequent visits.

Bente notes that it was at about age three that doctors told her parents that she would probably die of infection and breathing problems before she was five years old. Nevertheless, her parents brought her up at home and she was "mainstreamed" through school and into a job as a clerk in a hospital. Listen to her words in her second language, English, describing what happened to her next.

> I had never been sick with an infection or had breathing problems before I was 24 years old but then I suddenly caught a cold. I did not have muscle power enough to cough and during a few days I got a pneumonia, came to the intensive ward where they treated me with a respirator and a tube through the nose for two or three weeks.
>
> After a month I began to work again but I did not feel well. It was almost impossible to wake up in the morning, I had a headache, I could not eat because I felt sick, I could not concentrate on anything,

> I fell asleep while I was talking, my periods stopped, my hair fell off, and I got incontinent. I was tired to the bone but I could not sleep because of nightmares of the dead.
>
> For all these symptoms I got a lot of medicine. I got medicine for the blood pressure which was high because of the breathing problem, medicine to make it easier to breathe, for the heart, medicine for my sickness and other kinds of medicine that I cannot remember any longer.
>
> During that year I was treated with a respirator and a nasal tube four times about fourteen days each. I was at the hospital most of that year. The symptoms came sooner and sooner after the respirator treatments and much worse. At last I was unconscious. Nobody told me or my family at any time what was wrong and I did not know anything about a tracheostomy and a permanent respirator as a possibility for survival.

Note that Bente and her family were not involved at this time, either in receiving information on the options for medical treatments or in the choice of treatment.

> One day I woke up at another hospital with a tracheostomy (and with a ventilator) and after some weeks I felt that my body began to work again. It was a wonderful experience. I had been fired from my work because of too much illness and days off. Then I got the disablement pension from the county. I got no counseling about ventilator use and I did not know any ventilator users so I had to find out everything myself. I was so happy to get enough air and I felt that I could manage everything.
>
> When I later asked the doctors why they did not tell me about a tracheostomy and a permanent respirator, they answered that it had been difficult to find a solution for me. Some of the doctors thought that it was impossible to live a life of quality with a spinal atrophy and as a permanent respirator user. Other ones thought it was possible and wanted to give me the chance.

Again, note that Bente had had no part in making this critical life-or-death decision. To continue:

> I was afraid to breathe by myself because it had been so terrible an experience not to be able to breathe and I loved my respirator and the feeling of getting air enough without thinking about every breath, to sleep without nightmares of the dead, and to feel how my body began to work again. Using my respirator all the time I felt much better, had much more power and energy. I could talk loud and clear without

> getting tired and after one-and-a-half years in the hospital system, I felt that life was waiting for me again.

Thus, Bente was given the opportunity to live. We have to assume that her doctors were acting in what they considered her best interest. The critical question about quality of life with full-time ventilator use was answered by each doctor from his or her own personal perspective, rather than from Bente's perception of what constituted "quality of life." This is clearly a decision which must be based on the principle: Do unto others as *they* would have you do unto *them.* In this case: Do unto Bente as *she* would have you do unto *her.*

The next question, then, is, "What quality of life has Bente had since receiving her tracheostomy and ventilator?"

Gini Laurie recalled meeting Bente in Copenhagen at the Collective House, where many people with disabilities live. She asked Gini, "Do people with disabilities and ventilators really live independently in the community?" Gini encouraged her to try.

Since then, with Denmark's independent living policy, Bente has moved to her own apartment, and has helpers 24 hours a day. While the county pays their wages, Bente functions as their employer. She uses a battery-powered wheel chair, which also runs her ventilator. She proudly emphasizes that she has full responsibility for her life.

Again, in her words:

> I am active in the organizations and give lectures to doctors, nurses, and teachers on the psychological, social, and educational aspects of living with a disability. I plan courses, participate on panels about breathing problems, and work as a counselor for persons with muscular dystrophy and breathing problems.
>
> Besides giving lectures, I like very much to go around, like people without disability, to enjoy movies, theaters, exhibitions, restaurants, and jazz-houses. I like to travel and to find my limits. During my career as a respirator user I have found out that there are a lot of things you cannot do because of your physical disability *but nothing you cannot do because of your tracheostomy.*

In 1987, Bente came to the US funded by five foundations to study how persons with respiratory disabilities are treated here and to attend the GINI International Polio and Independent Living Conference. Her report is entitled, *Good Wind: A Report About the Treatment of and Attitudes Toward Respirator Handicapped Persons in the USA.* She drove from the East Coast to the West Coast, and three photographs from her trip stand out. The first is of her floating in a swimming pool, with her helper using an air bag on her trachea. The second is of her riding a ski lift up a mountainside with her helper sitting next to her, again using the air bag. The third—which epitomizes to me her zest for life—is of her sitting on a stone wall on the edge of the Grand Canyon, with her feet hanging over and her helper holding on to her while Bente leans forward to look down.

In Bente's last letter to me, she was looking forward to going to Moscow to talk about the Danish disability organization. "I haven't been there yet," she said.

The question regarding quality of life and the use of a ventilator must be left for you to answer for yourself. Clearly, Bente has answered it in the affirmative. I might add that I have answered in the affirmative, as well, but I must admit my own bias, since as a result of polio I have used a ventilator and other breathing aids for sleeping for 35 years.

What are the implications of Bente's story? They are many, but three stand out. First, it is important that adequate information and options are given to each disabled person. Bente's ignorance of her options nearly cost her her life.

Second, the rights of individuals to make choices and control their own lives must always be considered.

Finally, "quality of life" is a phenomonological concept, and can not be defined by one person for another.

19

A 35-YEAR PERSPECTIVE ON THE UTILIZATION OF MECHANICAL VENTILATION AS EXPERIENCED BY THE AUTHOR

Ira W. Holland

GENERAL INTRODUCTION

In August 1955, at the age of 15, while employed as a counselor at a summer camp on Cape Cod, Massachusetts, I was disabled as the result of polio. The last of the polio epidemics struck Boston during the latter part of that summer; hundreds died or were disabled only a few weeks prior to the availability of Dr. Salk's vaccine. Two young campers became ill within a few days of entering the camp. My exposure to these children while working with them evidently exposed me to the polio virus.

ONSET ACUTE STAGE

Within one week I became acutely ill. My inability to walk, bouts of nausea, and muscle spasms accompanied by a high fever resulted in my being transported by ambulance from the camp to a local hospital on the Cape. A spinal tap performed at the hospital confirmed the diagnosis of polio, and I was transferred to Haynes Memorial Hospital in Boston, Massachusetts.

Upon admission to Haynes Memorial, I had great difficulty breathing, which necessitated my being placed into an Emerson iron lung. As the tank was sealed, I experienced the extraordinary relief of air rushing to fill my lungs after laboring for so many hours to inhale barely enough to stay alive. I do not recall the next two weeks but remember waking to find myself transformed from a trim, active, athletic teenager to a quadriplegic, with no free breathing time, who was only able to speak in the manner that is permitted by any mechanically assisted device. The severe pain and spasms which tore through my back and limbs were alleviated, to some extent, by the application of moist hot packs.

When I woke into this nightmare, my parents were standing close by, masks covering their faces and sterile gowns their bodies. Their attempts to comfort me were somehow lost in the terror that gripped me. My food was mashed and offered to me on a spoon. I was told by a young resident, Dr. Edward R. Ritvo, to swallow so as not to aspirate my food. My bowels and kidneys were accommodated with urinal and bedpans that were inserted through a small port that opened on the side of the tank. My bath, my linen change, and my unbearable need to flex my arms and legs were accomplished by nurses who thrust their arms through sponge-encircled portholes so as not to interrupt my breathing. I was certain I would die at any time. Thirty iron lungs lined both sides of the large Infectious Disease Ward at Haynes. Throughout the next few months, I was witness to other patients dying. Two patients opposite my tank respirator died and were removed while in their machines. The pretense of maintaining life was continued by the staff as the tank respirators were "hand pumped" while the patients were moved elsewhere.

My tank respirator was opened each day to see if I could "breath on my own." These attempts were to no avail. I would try desperately to fill my lungs, but after a minute or two I felt that I would suffocate and it was apparent that my breathing would remain dependent on the ventilator. Three months elapsed, during which my family visited on frequent trips from New York. I was both frightened and embarrassed at my complete dependence upon others to accomplish every physical need. My continued reliance upon the Emerson iron lung was a source of extraordinary concern. I began to think there would be no future if I remained within this device.

By this time it was early fall. Many of the patients with whom I had spoken had died. I wanted very much to get out alive.

Dr. Ritvo spoke with me for many hours, particularly in the evenings, when the unit was relatively quiet. He told me about the existence of other breathing devices and that this hospital could offer nothing in the way of rehabilitation. He said he and one of my favorite nurses would accompany me back to New York City.

REHABILITATIVE PROCESS

In November 1955 I was transferred, while in the iron lung, by means of a large moving truck with a generator attached, to Goldwater Memorial Hospital on Roosevelt Island. After a nine-hour ordeal that encompassed the discomfort of travel within the body of an iron lung, police escorts through four states, the roar of the generator, and my humiliation at being met by my parents and younger brother, who were surrounded by a mob of newspaper and camera people at the entrance to the hospital, I was "unloaded" at the Goldwater Memorial Hospital Respiratory Rehabilitation Center, which was at the time part of the March of Dimes network of Polio Respiratory Rehabilitation Centers. Within the next 30 minutes I was quickly transferred from the iron lung that had been my "home" for the past three months, into another tank respirator, so that my initial ventilator could be returned to the Boston hospital. In the process of transfer I had the first glimpse of my now atrophied body. I was startled at the sight of myself. In fact, it was as though I was looking at another body. The transformation to "quadriplegic" was now somehow complete. I could neither move nor breathe; my very life depended upon that large yellow machine. My anxiety level was at its highest point. Though a relatively brief period of time had elapsed, it seemed to me that I had been living this unreal experience for longer than three months.

I was met by a group of young physicians and nurses at Goldwater Hospital and was told that the Rehabilitation Center was the next step in the process of learning to live as a disabled person. They explained that the center worked with many others who had a ventilator dependency and that in time I would come to know these patients and share experiences.

The rehabilitative process had begun, and during the next three months I was weaned from the tank to the chest piece or curiass. I had begun to spend my days on a bed and to be lifted by two or three people to be returned to the "lung" for sleeping. At this point, more than seven months had elapsed, and I still had no free breathing time. My ability to properly ventilate on the Monaghan chest piece did continue to improve, to the point that I was able to be free of the iron lung.

During the next two months I was able to sit in a manual wheel chair at bedside while using the Monaghan negative pressure chest piece. The ventilator, which provided power to my shell, was the Monaghan Universal. The Universal is a large bedside console to which I was connected through the use of a five-foot hose.

My initial ventures outside the hospital incorporated the use of a cumbersome "portable" ventilator which was manufactured by J. J. Monaghan. The battery packs were 24 volt and required two very strong people to lift them. I had begun to use IPPV shortly after its introduction by Conatech-Huxley. The advent of IPPV permitted me to bathe and dress more easily. I was also able to remove the chest piece for a number of hours, thus giving rest to my skin surface.

As the rehabilitation process progressed, I slowly began to make emotional and psychological adjustments to this radical transformation from able-bodied to completely dependent. My meeting and speaking with other patients at the rehabilitation center served a very positive purpose. I was able to discuss my anxieties, my concerns, my fears regarding the future with people who were similarly disabled. I became close friends with a few other teenage young men. Over the period of the next ten years, my closest friend was Bruce. Bruce and I literally grew up together. We lived through our adolescence, completed high school, experimented with liquor, cigarettes, and girl friends. We learned that people who are dependent upon a ventilator can get drunk and feel just as sick as anyone else, that cigarettes can make breathing almost impossible if you have difficulty in the first place, and that it was very nice to have girls around to talk with, to hug, and to try all the things that any young person would want to experience. We spoke of parents, of brothers and sisters, of religion, and why God had done this. The period of sharing with Bruce, who was a year younger than I and who used virtually the same respiratory equipment, was invaluable to my emotional stability.

My ventilator dependency was becoming more a part of my reality. My awareness of the inherent risks and threats to my life as a result of my dependency were becoming more apparent. I was concerned with the threat of colds; I had become ill a few times and had to return briefly to the iron lung to recuperate. I was determined to continue using the ventilators that became available as new technology continued to improve this type of equipment.

With the introduction of the pneumbelt in the early 1960s, I found that I could achieve a much higher degree of mobility by using the belt in conjunction with the Huxley Multi-Lung while sitting in the chair. The pneumobelt permitted me more comfort than the chest piece and was aesthetically pleasing, as it could be worn under my clothes. So I established a ventilator combination that would be suitable for almost 20 years. The curiass was satisfactory for sleeping and the pneumobelt for mobility in the chair.

My activities were enhanced to an appreciable extent in 1968, when I received my first breath-controled power wheelchair. Thompson Respiration Products had introduced the small black "Bantam" ventilator, which could be mounted on the back of the chair and powered by a 12-volt battery. It was at this point that I was able to enter Long Island University in 1968.

LIVING WITHIN AN INSTITUTION

During the period of my six years of study at Long Island University, I continued to live at Goldwater Memorial Hospital, whose respiratory center had been opened in 1954 by the March of Dimes "National Foundation for Infantile Paralysis." March of Dimes funding was phased out in 1963 and the center operated as the New York Regional Respiratory Center, with funding from New York City. In 1979, the center changed its name to the Howard A. Rusk Respiratory Rehabilitation Center.

The experience of being able to attend a university, to participate in courses, to meet people, and to take responsibility for completing a program of study, was of significant importance. The small portable ventilators of this period provided me with a new sense of freedom. I was not tied to an AC outlet, and though the batteries were heavy and power consumption was high, I was able to make brief excursions into the world outside the hospital.

I remember clearly that at this point I became quite nervous. I realized that I was "at risk." I began to think about my ventilator malfunctioning. Though I had learned to frog breathe for a short while, I felt very vulnerable. My sense of accomplishment at college was an important stimulus. I wanted to complete my course of study, and so I came to terms with my apprehension. My "coming to terms" really means that I continued to reassess the risks against wanting to accomplish something of significance. I think that this process continues as long as one is a ventilator dependent person. There are periods when you focus, perhaps only for a very short time, on the fact that your life is tied to a ventilator. However, I would not have done anything differently, and I am pleased and proud that I have been able to direct my feelings toward that from which I get the most satisfaction, regardless of the risk.

Dr. Augusta Alba, who was initially a resident on the respiratory service, was now director of the Respiratory Rehabilitation Service at Goldwater. Dr. Alba's "team" of nurses, physicians, physical therapists, occupational therapists, respiratory therapists, and psychologists helped me find some structure within my uncertain existence. I wanted to leave the institution, but I was not clear as to what direction to take. My ventilator dependency was a primary concern to me. As for being discharged, it was difficult to envision living apart from the safe environment the hospital offered. As I continued to work with the rehabilitation team, a sense of confidence began to develop within me.

I graduated from Long Island University in 1973 and was ecstatic at the fact that I had actually completed this venture. I felt determined to continue, to leave the hospital and become involved in a productive pursuit, though I was not certain of my capabilities.

DISCHARGE PROCESS

I applied to St. John's Law School in 1974, after having scored reasonably well on the LSAT. I seriously considered a career in law but decided that first I wanted to leave the hospital and establish myself in my own home. In 1975 the Urban Development Corporation (UDC) completed the first phase of the Roosevelt Island apartment complex. I had worked for three years on a committee which had met with representatives of UDC and the Roosevelt Island Development Corporation (RIDC). The group's purpose was to make UDC and RIDC aware of the needs of the severely disabled population that would be living in some of its apartments. We spoke at length about accessibility, curb cuts, accessible buses (there is a small fleet of buses that operates on the island). We also addressed the issue of people who were ventilator dependent. UDC and RIDC were sensitive to the needs of the disabled population and took special care to know which apartments were occupied by people with ventilators so that they could assist them if electrical disruption were to present a problem. At this point in my life, I felt that the availability of an apartment on Roosevelt Island was the next logical step.

Dr. Alba's rehabilitation team worked with me to prepare me for discharge. An affiliation with a respiratory home care company was made, proper equipment was placed in my apartment, and all necessary supplies were delivered. I spent one last sleepless night at Goldwater Memorial Hospital on April 21, 1976. I lay awake wondering how my plans would work out. Would my home attendants arrive on time? Would they stay long enough for me to set myself up at home? There were many unanswered questions, but on the morning of April 22, 1976, with the assistance of some close friends (and a great deal of anxiety), I took the enormous step back into the community. I was re-entering a world that I had left 21 years earlier. At the age of 36, I was going home to live independently. I was still 24-hour ventilator dependent, although I had learned glossopharyngeal "frog" breathing. I was able to frog breathe for a period of two hours, which gave me sufficient time to transfer comfortably from bed to chair, and I always carried a second ventilator with me. This limited free time permitted me to switch the ventilators if one malfunctioned. My home attendants were recruited through a newspaper advertisement and were trained initially at Goldwater Memorial Hospital. They were thoroughly trained as regards assistive coughing, percussion, and the use of portable ventilators. More importantly, perhaps, I trained my attendants as regards my personal needs and how I wished to be taken care of, so that I might be functional, comfortable, and confident. I now had a place to live apart from a hospital bed and people who could assist me in a manner that was comfortable and compatible with my life style.

The discharge process was not without its problems. A power failure struck the Northeast shortly after I set up residence, and I learned how to deal effectively with a 14-hour loss of electric power. After emerging from that crisis, I felt much more certain about handling other possible emergencies. I was learning how to think and act quickly with the people who assisted me.

ESTABLISHING A LIFESTYLE IN THE COMMUNITY

The home care program that existed in New York City was in the process of evolving into a new format of service provision. Previously the city had operated the entire package. This was to be changed into a system that used not-for-profit corporations to provide home attendant services.

The prospect of not being able to hire my own home attendants and having a stranger sent into my own home was sufficient motivation for me to begin working with friends and colleagues to establish a home care agency. Our objective was to hire, train, and otherwise employ attendants compatible with our individual needs, and so Concepts of Independence, Inc., was conceived. It took two years and many hundreds of meetings with the state and city before Concepts was awarded its first contract in 1980. Concepts of Independence, Inc., began business with a staff of five people and a client census of twenty. Our initial contract provided $110,000. In the next ten years, we grew considerably. Our office staff is now comprised of ten people, our client census is at 300, and our current contract stands at $13 million. I am most pleased that as vice president of Concepts I have had the opportunity and pleasure to work closely with our president, board of directors, and staff to enable us to grow to this significant point.

The initial home care provider of ventilators went into bankruptcy after two years, and it was necessary for us to become affiliated with a second company. By this point my familiarity with ventilators had become rather extensive. I began working as a consultant to Thompson Respiration Products, Inc., in 1978. I prepared reports on new equipment and spoke with physicians, therapists, and ventilator-dependent people regarding the performance of current equipment and the need for revision.

I decided to present myself to the second home care company as a consultant. Paramedical Specialties, Inc., hired me in 1979, and I continued to work with them in the areas of discharge planning, ventilator applications, and inservice training.

In 1980, I had an upper respiratory infection that necessitated my returning to Goldwater Memorial Hospital, so I could use an iron lung, since my curiass was inadequate for ventilation. In fact, I had become aware that the chest piece was no longer compatible with proper ventilation a few months prior to my return. After recovering from my cold, I spoke with Dr. Alba regarding alternative ventilatory methods. She recommended that I be tested on the Puritan Bennett Lip Seal with velcro straps. This device proved to be satisfactory, and I have continued to use it in conjunction with the Puritan Bennett Maxivent for sleeping.

In 1983 Thompson Respiration Products was acquired by the Puritan Bennett corporation. Consequently, I have been a consultant to the Portable Ventilator Division of the Puritan Bennett Corporation for the past seven years. I have found the work both challenging and rewarding. I have had the opportunity to work with key people in this multinational manufacturer of ventilators. My activities involve the preparation of reports on equipment from my standpoint as one who has been ventilator-dependent for more than three decades. Through Puritan Bennett, my insights and expertise regarding the concerns of ventilator-dependent patients are shared with physicians, therapists, patients, and families. I am pleased that I am able to contribute to Puritan Bennett in a manner that enables them to produce a quality product directed at the specific needs of the ventilator-dependent patient. Many of my discussions and reports pertain to the improvement of portable ventilators and the further enhancement of the next generation so they better serve a growing population of users.

In similar fashion, my work with Paramedical Specialties, Inc., took a new direction with their acquisition first by Healthdyne, Inc., and more recently by the Glasrock Home Health Care Corporation. As a consultant to Glasrock, a major home health care provider, I work with ventilator-dependent patients who are ready for discharge and will need support services when they move into the community. I act as a liaison between the hospital, the patient, and Glasrock representatives, thus ensuring a smooth and uninterrupted flow of service and information. Many ventilator-dependent patients feel a greater sense of security about returning home if they work with someone who is similarly dependent. My services have often made a difference in the patient's ability to accept discharge as a viable alternative.

The ability to work and to make a significant and meaningful contribution is as important to a person who is disabled and ventilator dependent as it is to any other person.

I switched from the pressure regulated Thompson GS/GT to the Puritan Bennett M25B in 1982. As my activities increased, I began to find that the pressure regulated ventilators were not energy efficient. I am able to operate the M25B for 14 hours as compared to a relatively short six hours of operating time with the pressure regulated GS/GT ventilators. The GS/GT ventilators were not reliable to the same degree that the volume regulated devices are, and their imminent obsolescence made repairs much more difficult.

The M25B was used on my power chair in conjunction with the Puritan Bennett pneumobelt, which I have now used for more than 25 years. It remains comfortable and viable. In January 1989 I began using the Puritan Bennett Companion 2500 in place of the M25B. The Companion 2500 replaces the M25B, and I have found that the improved technology offers a higher degree of reliability and that it is easier for me to have my caregivers establish ventilator settings with this unit.

Since living independently in my apartment, I have hired a number of replacement home attendants. On average, most of them have remained with me for four to five years. The hiring of a home attendant who is compatible and sensitive to my needs is one of the most crucial aspects in a successful community living experience. In my opinion, the more complex a home care process, the more difficult it is to remain dependent upon family for the provision of home care services. I believe that the family is too emotionally involved with the disabled individual to be able to deal objectively with problems as they arise or to help find realistic solutions. Overall, a good home attendant will assist the ventilator dependent person to live as independently as is reasonably possible. I am, of course, assuming that the person is capable of self-direction.

Clothing and food must be shopped for, the house must be kept orderly, meals must be planned. If equipment requires repair, whether it is a wheelchair, a refrigerator, or the ventilator, we all must know who should be called. Transportation with a reliable carrier to and from my work, meetings, public-speaking engagements, and recreational pursuits must be arranged.

A ventilator dependent person is not in a position to be left alone for an extended period of time; clear thinking and planning with both friends and reliable employees are the keystones to success in this crucial area.

When a ventilator dependent person, like myself, must depend upon a caregiver for every aspect of personal care, it is imperative that the attendant understand clearly the responsibilities they are assuming. I feel that I have been careful in hiring attendants, and as a result I have been reasonably fortunate. Most of my caregivers have become much more to me than employees.

Meeting people, establishing relationships, going out for dinner, attending concerts, going on vacation; these are all part of a full life. Certainly, a full life is the goal of any of us, disabled, ventilator dependent, or able-bodied.

SETTING PRIORITIES AND GOALS

Thirty-five years have elapsed since I entered the iron lung in Boston in August 1955. The growth process has been accelerated by my almost insatiable desire to accomplish as much as I possibly can. Initially, I remember asking how long somebody like me would live. Five or ten years, I was told. After reaching that point, I asked again, and I remember being told that most people in my condition live for about 20 years. It was then that I stopped asking. I feel I have accomplished far more than I ever believed possible. I am deeply satisfied with my work and with my relationships. There are always problems to be solved, always some crisis to respond to, always an innumerable number of tasks, calls, people, and reports that need responding to. I honestly find that there are not enough hours to do all that is to be done.

Last October, I celebrated my fiftieth birthday. What an unimaginable milestone, when I look back to my arrival at Goldwater Memorial Hospital in 1955. I had a birthday party and invited some 40 friends and colleagues, people that I love. I had returned six weeks earlier from a wonderful vacation on Cape Cod with two dear friends, and while there I visited the hospital where it all began 35 years ago. In many respects, it seems a lifetime away.

The accomplishments that can and are being made by ventilator dependent people in today's world are both startling and real. I am pleased and proud to know many others like myself who are functional, productive people, living full and active lives. The possibilities are endless. There are problems that I share with those who do not use ventilators, and there are problems I must solve myself. The process goes on. Each of us has but one opportunity, and I am determined to make the most of it. People have asked me to tell them which year I consider the most fulfilling, what period of my life I feel reflects my most extensive accomplishment. I would say that this present period is the most deeply satisfying.

A ventilator-dependent person should be given every opportunity to have access to today's technology. If the decision is made to make a ventilator available to a patient, a commitment to that patient must be part of the offer. The commitment must include the opportunity for the individual to access whatever essential services are necessary to insure that his or her quality of life will be the highest possible. To make a ventilator available to a person who is vegetative is of questionable value, and to deny support services to a patient who is aware and who has the potential to be functional is a disservice. The ventilators of the 1990s are in every respect assistive devices. They are less intrusive, more reliable, and quieter than any similar mechanical device previously devised. Certainly, today's ventilators have evolved through many generations to a point where a capable person who is dependent upon a ventilator has a real opportunity to lead a full and productive life.

I would like to say that I am grateful that mechanical ventilation and the necessary medical expertise was made available to me 35 years ago. I am realistic about my life as a ventilator-dependent person. I think I am a good example for offering mechanical ventilation to people who may benefit from it. It is certainly a tool to be used with discretion.

20

OPTIONS FOR LIVING AND DYING IN AMYOTROPHIC LATERAL SCLEROSIS

Augusta Alba, M.D.

A hospital caring for long-term patients, with a respiratory rehabilitation center for neuromuscular disorders, has had more than 30 years experience in the management of the ALS patient who is a ventilator user. A client may elect to remain at home until a critical illness or other crisis supervenes. He or she may remain at home with little or no help or with as much ancillary help as can be afforded. In either instance, when the client becomes critically ill, he or his family must decide whether to rush him to a local emergency room where intubation and mechanical ventilation will be instituted, or to allow him to die at home. Whatever the decision, it should have been discussed far in advance and frequently reviewed by the decision makers. If the patient is taken to a hospital, he or she may survive an intercurrent illness and elect to return home with or without the need for ventilator support.

The following cases (1) illustrate ongoing decision making by clients and their families where the client lives at home.

CASE 1

A hard-working widower and junkyard owner was in his sixties when it was discovered he had ALS. He had one son living within 20 minutes of his home, who checked on him. He sought no further help. He continued working until he could no longer crawl up the flight of stairs to his apartment and fell frequently. One year later he was found in a moribund state. He was rushed to a local hospital where he was resuscitated, intubated, and placed on mechanical ventilation. Weeks went by before he died.

CASE 2

A businessman developed ALS in the mid-1980s. His wife is a psychiatrist. Together they decided to have him cared for at home, with RNs around the clock. Her insurance covered this type of care for catastrophic illness. Gradually, his condition deteriorated. He permitted a gastrotomy tube. His speech became unintelligible. He could no longer stand, but insisted on being dragged out of bed with his body weight hanging from his armpits so that he could use the commode. He vacillated between wanting to go to the hospital for a tracheostomy and remaining at home without it. He feared his wife was trying to kill him. With caution, she gave him sleeping capsules at night for his marked insomnia and an antidepressant during the day under his physician's direction. He refused a ventilator at home but accepted oxygen and IPPB treatments. These treatments gradually increased in frequency to the extent that during the day he was using the machine as a ventilator by mouth. He died peacefully in his sleep more than one year after his death had been considered a certainty. His wife's courage and finances were nearly exhausted at the time; his two daughters had become distraught and spent much of their time out of the home.

CASE 3

ALS started in this patient, a writer, like "upside down polio," with involvement of the respiratory muscles, upper trunk, and arms before the legs. He adapted quickly to MIPPV and used it with a lipseal at night. He made a decision, with the help of his wife, to die at such time as he was no longer able to communicate. He did not want a tracheostomy. He lived 15 months on a ventilator. During that time he commuted briefly to Boston for treatment with an experimental drug. He bagged himself for artificial ventilation on the plane by using his foot with a compressible manual resuscitator. On one occasion, he developed acute bronchopneumonia and could not handle the secretions. He elected to be intubated during the course of this illness. The endotracheal tube was removed in less than one month and he returned to using MIPPV. Months later, when he had just completed an article for publication, he developed a minor upper respiratory infection and lost his ability to swallow. Although he was intent on dying at home, he could not bear to have his wife see his suffering. He agreed to hospitalization at an acute care hospital, where he was placed in an iron lung and treated for aspiration pneumonia. His wishes were honored: he was not intubated or tracheostomized. He died two weeks later.

A patient, after admission to an acute care hospital, may find that alternative placement is more feasible. By various means, the stay at the acute hospital may be extended for months or even years. More commonly, the patient will be transferred to a long-term care hospital or a skilled nursing facility. At the long-term care facility, the patient may have borderline respiratory function adequate for survival and may elect to use no form of assisted ventilation. He or she may elect to use noninvasive ventilation: combinations of noninvasive intermittent positive pressure ventilation (mouth, nasal, or nasal/mouth interfaces), and body ventilators (pneumobelt, cuirass, iron lung). He may accept a tracheostomy with tracheal intermittent positive pressure ventilation. The need for mechanical ventilation will be complete either by the time of admission or will increase to fulltime support over a period of months or years. The patient living in an institution must be provided with a satisfactory lifestyle. Support groups, friends, family, TV and radio, use of augumentative communication devices and a motorized wheelchair, recreational events, and computer access are some of the factors that make life worth living.

The following cases illustrate ongoing decision making in an institution.

CASE 4

A female ALS patient in her seventies had lived in a long-term-care hospital for three years on MIPPV around the clock, in spite of her being edentulous. She had been able to use a motorized chair. Her condition then deteriorated to the point that she could no longer use the MIPPV or the chair. She chose to remain alive on mechanical ventilation via TIPPV, and a tracheostomy was performed. She spent the next two years of her life in bed with a TV and a radio, some family and friends as visitors, until her death.

CASE 5

An elderly male patient with ALS is completely ventilator-dependent, unable to move except for his eyelids and eyeballs. He has had recurrent intercurrent illnesses that have been life-threatening and have required extended stays in the special care unit. A psychiatrist interviewed him recently with the help of the speech pathologist, who has expertise in alternate communication methods, and was surprised by his eye-blink answers to her questions. She posed the question of resuscitation in at least three different ways and, in spite of his state of bodily imprisonment, he answered her repeated questions regarding resuscitation in the affirmative.

Since ALS is considered a terminal illness, a patient should be encouraged to write a living will as early in the course of hospitalization as possible. A Bioethics Committee, with participation of the key personnel treating the client, including the physician, psychiatrist, patient representative, chaplain, psychologist, speech pathologist, social worker, and nursing staff, with participation of the client and/or family, should meet promptly to endorse the living will. The committee should meet throughout the client's stay at the institution, as the need arises. A do-not-resuscitate (DNR) order can be requested by the client if he is considered competent by his caregivers, by the family if he is not competent, or by the treating physicians if there is no family. In a long-term care setting, a DNR is renewed every 30 days, when all other medical orders are renewed. The client's wishes are reaffirmed whenever the order is renewed, and documentation is placed in the chart. The family may write a declaration of intent if the client is not competent. However, they are made aware that the hospital is not legally bound to follow their requests. After thorough input from legal counsel, both for the client and the institution, the declaration of intent is endorsed by the Bioethics Committee, if it is reasonable.

The following case illustrates the use of a living will.

CASE 6

A retired captain in the New York City police force was quadriplegic and completely ventilator-dependent by TIPPV when he entered a long-term care hospital ventilator center. On a frequent basis, his friends on the police force arranged for him to go home with his motorized wheelchair for a day. He participated in the poetry club at the hospital. He arranged a living will, in which he requested no artificial feedings, including no gastrotomy tube. He expressed a wish to die when he could no longer swallow. His swallowing began to fail in November of the year that the case of a young woman with cerebral palsy, who wanted a hospital in California to permit her to starve herself to death, was brought to court. The court decided that the hospital did not have to do this. Our patient gradually became able to eat less and less through January of the following year. The hospital authorities became alarmed at his slow starvation, even though they had endorsed his living will. However, by the time they considered ordering the medical staff to feed him, the client had developed severe metabolic acidosis, could be treated only with intravenous fluids, slipped into a coma, and quietly died. He had written a poem one year earlier, describing the horror of having to remain alive in a body that no longer responded to his needs.

After an indeterminate period of time at the institution, a patient and his or her family may request the patient's discharge and return home in order for him to be disconnected from the ventilator. The patient, if competent, may request to be disconnected from the ventilator at the hospital in a humane fashion.

The following case illustrates the use of a living will to request being disconnected from the ventilator.

CASE 7

This case involves a male in his late seventies who came to the ventilator center as a quadriplegic, completely dependent on a ventilator via TIPPV, and with a gastrotomy for feeding. Upper extremity function was minimal and was gradually lost. He retained some ability to speak. His well-meaning wife agonized over his bodily functions. Together they made the decision to disconnect his ventilator. He had written a living will with the help of an augmentative communication device. Two adult children, both professionals, and his wife refused to take him home so he could be disconnected. Ultimately, the hospital agreed to help. He was moved to a private room. The nursing staff was thoroughly briefed concerning his wishes. His wife agreed to disconnect the ventilator, and one of the physicians agreed to give him an intravenous sedative. His wife, children, a chaplain, and close friends were to be there. The patient died three days before his planned demise.

Now we will discuss issues that are often raised with the Bioethics Committee by patients or families. Clients have refused intubation, tracheostomy, gastrotomy, artificial ventilation, CPR, oxygen, antibiotics and other medications to prolong life, surgery, and transfer to a special care unit or another hospital. Most have accepted mechanical ventilation and gastrotomy by the time they are transferred to a long-term-care hospital. Most want the ventilator disconnected and feeding by gastrotomy tube stopped if an irreversible mental condition occurs and they can no longer participate in decision making. Whenever families write a Declaration of Intent, the Bioethics Committee must carefully check to see that the client is not capable of decision making or of any reliable communication. Unless there is written evidence that the patient did not want what is considered good medical care before he became incompetent, we cannot accept the family's request not to provide reasonable medical care.

Patients generally want as much pain medication as is needed. Even in the most advanced condition, they have asked for new methods of treatment. L-threonine was given to several of them in the past three years. One benefitted when her spasticity and pain, her major source of suffering, subsided. Families have also requested medications that have not been shown to be effective, such as dl-phenylalanine for pain and calcium EAP form of colamine phosphate, a mineral transporter said to protect cells against autoimmune attack. In these instances our neurological staff has not agreed to give the medications.

In conclusion, it must be realized that the options for living and dying with ALS are in a constant state of flux, evolving with the progression of the illness. It requires infinite patience and compassion on the part of caregivers to provide a dignified, warm, and understanding environment when mounting complications and death greet them on a daily basis in their care of these courageous people. [1]

NOTES

1. Some of this material was presented at the Fifth International Post-Polio Conference and Symposium on Living Independently with Severe Disability, June 1989. It has been reproduced here with the permission of the Gazette International Networking Institute, 4502 Maryland Avenue, St. Louis, Missouri 63108.

21

IMPACT ON THE FAMILY

Margaret Mikol

One series of items attempted to gain a sense of how the demands of home care affected the daily life of the patient's family. In this area, it is impossible to separate the answers to the questions in the survey from the interviews. Each family had a unique story, and the survey only provided a forum to start the families describing their experiences in caring for their child. It is in this area that the interview data is the richest.

Perhaps the greatest impact of a child's disability is when the family must be separated because of the child's care needs. In the study group, 17 percent of the children had been placed out of the home at some time. A measure of the pressure on the families can be seen in the fact that 27 percent of them had considered out-of-home placement for their child. It is important to note that this out-of-home placement means placement in an institution, nursing home, or community group home, and does not include time spent in acute care hospitals or temporary respite. In the area of employment, 31 percent of the prime caregivers work out of the home at least part of the time. During the last year, all of these individuals had to take some time off work to care for their children. Eighty percent had to take time off at least once a month. Additionally, 44 percent of the respondents indicated that a spouse or other adults in the home had to take time off from work. One-third of these had to take time off at least once a month.

A group of what might be called the "opportunity costs" are associated with home care: major changes in life style, physical environment, daily routine, or opportunities for personal development that have been influenced by the care needs of the child with special needs.

An example of an opportunity cost is seen in the 73 percent of respondents who said their childs' disability had effected where the family lived. When we look at the interview follow-up to this question, we find the cost takes three forms: 1) some families consciously chose to live in an area where they thought there were good services—the New York Metropolitan area; 2) some families chose to live in a neighborhood close to the hospital or clinic that would treat their child; and 3) many families found the expenses associated with the care of their child either made it impossible for them to move into the kind of housing they wanted or forced them to sell a home and live in an apartment or less expensive house.

In reviewing the families' comments that accompany their responses to the list of opportunity costs, it becomes evident that the list of categories, although useful to the researcher, does not capture the impact which the child's needs often have on the family. As in the case below, merely saying that the child's disability influenced where the family lived hardly captures the reality.

> Mom quit work; has to be home at all times. They live in a home with four generations of the family to cut down costs and to care for aging parents and grandmother. They cannot afford to live elsewhere because of Jim's expenses. Even with this proximity Mom cannot spend enough time with her dying mother because of Jim's care needs. The family's at the mercy of fifteen different systems. They cannot fix or sell house because of the financial stress.

In addition to some of the obvious costs of care which have modified their lifestyle, a number of families speak of more subtle factors at work within their homes. Margie's family's cultural differences made them aware that various professionals with different value systems were always "evaluating" them.

> Knowing that Margie still needs a lot of nursing but it is so invasive. We do not seem to spend enough time as a family. It is bad always having therapists and nurses around. They do not understand what a "big Spanish" family looks like. We yell, we shout, we laugh, we hug—we are just a typical family. We need better and more discreet nurses. Some of our nurses work on other home cases and they speak about them so they must be speaking about us.

The global transformation which the families experience usually begins at birth or shortly thereafter, when the child's condition becomes evident. Many families tell similar stories of being overwhelmed by the experience. This is often intensified in the hospital context and by the demeanor of the professionals at birth. Families tell of professionals dealing with them in a cold, detached manner that contributed to the confusion they were already feeling. Some recount a sense of being, or even accusations that they are, to blame for their child's condition. The attitude of the immediate and extended family is often formed by this initial negative experience. In many cases the family changes its attitude towards the child—but not always. The experience of Gini and her mother is illustrative.

> Mom had a long and difficult labor. The baby's deformities were visible at birth and the Ob-gyn. and pediatrician looked at Mom and said that it was her fault because she had smoked when she was pregnant. The condition is not related to that at all—it is a genetic defect that is inherited or a freak of nature. Mom was not shown the child for two days and was just told that the baby was in the neonatal unit. After two days the nurses came in and told her that babies get very well taken care of at institutions otherwise it gets too hard on the parents. She then brought Gini in. Mom cannot even describe her emotions or confusion. Mom thought about putting her up for adoption. The hospital suggested this and Gini's father said that Mom had to choose between him and Gini. Mom found out about the services she could get if she brought her home. Grandma went to visit a long term care home. Her reaction to this place impacted greatly on Mom's decision. The mom broke up with Gini's father more quickly since he will not get involved with the care of the child.

Just as Gini's grandmother's exposure to institutionalization influenced the family's decision to provide home care, so many other families recount similar reactions, which either strengthened or formed their resolve to take their child home.

> While in hospital, their son was on vent for twenty-four hours. Parents did not want to take child home on vent—especially twenty-four hours a day. Social worker and a nurse suggested Miller Memorial Hospital (a local long-term care facility), to institutionalize the child. The parents were overwhelmed due to the one year of hospitalization, trach, tube feeding and ventilator dependency. They were thinking of placing him in Miller Memorial until he could breathe on his own. On SKIP's advice they visited Miller Memorial before making a decision. Immediately after visit they called and stated that they would not under any circumstances place their son in such an environment. They were shocked at the lack of stimulation and care children received there and felt their son would not receive the stimulation and caring that he needed. Instead, they chose to take him home even if he had to be on a vent twenty-four hours a day. Very shortly after the hospital weaned him off the vent, so he only required it during the night while sleeping, the family could not understand why the staff at the hospital had recommended such a place as Miller Memorial for their son. After

all, even though he is ventilator-dependent, he is an active, alert child who needs a healthy, caring, and stimulating environment.

Once the initial shock is dealt with and the decision is made to care for the child at home, most of the families speak of being totally unprepared for the radical changes that follow. One family responded to the inquiries in this area with a stream of consciousness inventory of physical, social, and psychological changes that are associated with the care of their child.

> Ran tubes in walls for oxygen and bought a van—small eating trays—purchase stands—and closet space for supplies. We have borne all expenses and done most of it ourselves. Paper towels—peroxide—food—phone bills—travel expenses to Chicago—electricity—extra phones—intercoms. Total lifestyle change—no flexibility as far as coming and going. Oxygen has to be measured—nursing services are restricted to in home care and no privacy—we do not entertain as much.

Another parent's narrative of the effect that Jim has had on the life of his family also covers most of the bases. Particularly noteworthy is the emphasis on how Jim's needs have had an effect on his brother. This was a special area of concern in every case where the child with special care needs had siblings.

> I (Dad) can write a book on it (the changes in their life)—You lose all flexibility. The brother didn't have a normal 3rd and 4th year of childhood. He spent it in the hospital with his brother and he is very sensitive. The parents try to compensate. The family gets separated because they can't just get in the van and go. No spontaneity. Brother is too young but is starting to know the names of certain equipment and can help in a pinch. He often wants to just stay home with his brother. Mom can't seek outside employment because of Jim. Mom had to drop out of school. We are moving back to the city to be closer to the hospital—moving closer to friends, family and support. We cannot think about having another child. Jim is at home. Jim is striving towards being a typical kid —his brother loves him and is so glad he is home. Jim is happy and so adjusted. Mom feels all this made her a stronger person. It made our marriage stronger. Jim is a joy. Made the priorities clear—life is better defined.

The extensive list of the child's disabilities, complex care needs, daily crises, effects on the family lifestyle, and other factors related to providing home care which we have reviewed thus far are powerful data. No family exposed to these forces can avoid profound stress and major changes. Yet the effect of these lists and percentages are somewhat deceptive. What is missing here is some measure of the positive results of the decision to care for a child at home. The positive impact comes through only when we listen to the parents' stories.

The majority of families speak of the enormous improvement they witness in their child's physical and psychological condition once they come home as the most tangible affirmation of their decision to provide care at home. This is accompanied by an emerging awareness of their capacity and competence as parents. When we probed about some less concrete outcomes of home care, we heard families talk about getting to know their children as a person, seeing them as a contributing member of the family, experiencing a sense of togetherness, a growing sense of personal strength, the reordering of life's priorities, siblings learning to be caring people, and other factors not as easily quantified as pieces of special equipment .

One family characterized the positive effect of its decision to care for their daughter at home in terms of finally being able to accept her as their daughter.

> The family (Mom and Dad) felt enormous stress. And as they look back on their feelings they considered Sissy an extension of her equipment. During last winter their nursing (twenty-four hours per day) was cut back and the parents were obligated to provide the care. Mom feels like she thought she would have a nervous breakdown at first. Even though she was exhausted and nervous she realized she could meet the care demands—she started bonding with Sissy for the first time since her birth. She said that smoother transition to fewer hours of nursing would have been better, but she made it through the situation and she feels good. Now even though the financing problems have been resolved she schedules less nursing to spend more one on one time with Sissy. Mom feels that this is a very bad way to learn a good lesson.
>
> They have gotten through the tremendous fear of her imminent death because she is doing better and as a result have allowed themselves to see her as other than an extension of her equipment.

As the following excerpts from the interviews with Pete's adoptive mother and Morris's uncle testify, the need to see the patient as a child—a unique, growing human being—may be the positive outcome of these parents' experience. It is also clear from these and many other interviews that it is this awareness which gives the families the strength to endure all they must confront.

> Most stress and dissatisfaction comes from outside sources. Pete has been a joy (despite his problems) and I have never regretted my

> decision to adopt him. I have learned (and I am still learning) from him everyday, both as a professional and as a mother. Pete's excitement about life and learning despite his severe problems, despite his past, is remarkable. His achievements, emotionally, academically, artistically over the past three years are amazing, considering his hospitalization in the ICU for four and one-half years. Best of all Pete is a funny, bright, loving child who gets into lots of mischief to keep me busy, but who constantly makes me laugh (often at ourselves). Pete has enriched our family in a way that no one else could, and each of us has learned something about ourselves through him. Not one of us would trade a single hour with Pete for a winning lottery ticket. We're all very proud of him. Pete is the most loved member of his immediate and his extended family.

> His Uncle, just came in on the interview and says: "Morris is a spoiled great kid who we all have ruined." (We all laugh). "The little king, we call him. The only one he minds is Mom. He looks at the rest of us like we are nuts. He loves to tag along with me but I worry that he will fall asleep if I take him too far. It is funny how this little kid wraps people and gets them to do the things he wants them to do. Mom never lets any of us carry on like that — we would have had very sore backsides. She is funny too because she says she is hard on him, she is getting old and soft." Mom: "ALL RIGHT NOW!"

Many of the parents, particularly the mothers, speak of the experience of fighting for their child as totally reordering their value system and giving them a different perspective on their own competence. Charlene's and John's mothers make some of the strongest statements of this new growth in both self-awareness and social awareness.

> Mom has saved her life. Mom also feels that Charlene has saved her life and put things in order. Charlene has made Mom realize just what life means. Charlene has taught Mom about the practical application of health care. Patience—mom has learned—how to be frugal—keep a budget—self-reliance—independence—survival.

> John has taught his mother the beauty of the power of each human life. John has made Mom a more socially conscious person and given Mom the best sense of worth in her entire life. Has spurred Mom on to help others. John introduced Mom to God. He has helped Mom to understand unconditional love, he has sharpened Mom's compassion for all disabled people and advocacy efforts, (all people) none of us is without a disability. He enunciates the shape we are in as a society.

In summary, the families are very clear on the extensive costs that are associated with their decision to care for their own children at home. But, as a group, they are very clear on the dividends they are accruing.

> Her sister is limited in her activities because when Ryan gets sick they don't want her exposed to new infections. Ryan has chicken pox today and is doing quite well. Cynthia (her sister) still drinks from a bottle when she is more upset. When Ryan is sick she'll want to stay home. She is rough with Ryan when she is well. Cynthia once pointed out to Mom that she was the only one getting punished so Mom took note of this and now there's more equalized treatment. In addition, Dad is working two jobs to make ends meet. Now he will be stopping this fall. He had to do this for insurance purposes. Nevertheless, we have a beautiful, happy, well-adjusted child and an intact family. The interviewer notes at this point: Ryan is now at the sink spraying water over all of us which captures what she is all about.

22

VENTILATOR USERS, HOME CARE, AND INDEPENDENT LIVING

A Historical Perspective

Gini Laurie

INTRODUCTION

Gini often called polio the motif of her life. She was born in 1913, the first child of a "second" family after the 1912 polio epidemic in St. Louis took the lives of two sisters, severely disabled a brother, and mildly affected another sister.

When Gini's husband, Joe, was transferred to Cleveland in the late 1940s, it was only natural for her to volunteer at the Toomey Respiratory Pavilion during the polio epidemics of the 1950s. In 1958, she started the *Toomey j. Gazette,* a newsletter later to become the *Rehabilitation Gazette,* to help polio survivors keep in touch. The thirtieth anniversary edition of the *Gazette* contains articles by many of those survivors and is a perfect testimonial, that, yes, life with a ventilator can be good.

The *Gazette* grew into a worldwide information center and network of individuals with disabilities. Gini was the driving force behind the publication of *Handbook on the Late Effects of Poliomyelitis for Physicians and Survivors* and the catalyst for the international conferences on the late effects of polio. The *Gazette* became the umbrella organization for the International Polio Network and the International Ventilator Users Network.

As unofficial archivist for the independent living movement, Gini's unparalleled collection of books, papers, and letters attracted rehabilitation professionals, scholars, and individuals with disabilities from around the world. In the last few years, she travelled widely as an ambassador for all people with a disability, speaking about the history of the American independent living movement.

The following is her chapter entitled "Ventilator Users, Home Care, and Independent Living: An Historical Perspective."

In medical history, mechanical ventilation is a recent development. The first iron lung was developed in 1927 at Harvard University by Professor Phillip Drinker and Dr. Louis Shaw. Their first iron lung patient was a cat. They paralyzed its breathing and placed it in an airtight box with alternative air pressure from a vacuum cleaner motor. Two years later, Professor Drinker created the first iron lung for human beings.

The first person to live at home and travel extensively with a ventilator was Frederick Snite, Jr., the son of a wealthy Chicagoan. At age 25 he was disabled by respiratory polio in 1936 in Peking, China. At that time, there were only 222 iron lungs in the world and one just happened to be at the Peking Medical College for use with opium smokers.

Frederick stayed in that lung for over a year, then came home in it on a 21-day trip via truck, ocean liner and train. (His trans-Pacific party occupied 12 cabins and consisted of a physician, 7 Chinese nurses, a Chinese physiotherapist, two American nurses and his family.)

Frederick's life in a lung fascinated the American press—especially after he married and fathered three daughters.

He learned how to live independently. His biographer wrote, "He governed his own life. He made the decisions. He tackled and solved the problems. He gave the orders." Frederick lived in the lung at home from 1936 to 1954, when he died of cor pulmonale.

By 1949, there were 400 other respiratory polio survivors using ventilators in the U. S. who were not at home but in custodial care at over a hundred hospitals scattered around the country. They were funded by the National Foundation for Infantile Paralysis (the March of Dimes) which President Franklin Roosevelt had founded. The hospital charges for the 400 were so exorbitant that the March of Dimes initiated a study to find ways to reduce the cost. The study showed that it would be far more economical to move them to regional centers with multi-disciplinary professional teams.

This was done and, eventually, there were 16 polio respiratory and rehabilitation centers at the teaching hospitals of 16 medical schools, ranging in size from 15 to 160 patients.

The first two centers were set up in Boston and Houston in 1950. The lifespan of most of the centers was less than a decade (the average was six years), but their impact on physical medicine, independent living, and vocational rehabilitation of ventilator users, and other individuals with severe disabilities, was tremendous.

The timing of the opening of the centers was propitious because they were in place just in time for the devastating polio epidemics of the early 1950s in which so many young adults were disabled by respiratory paralysis.

During those terror-ridden epidemic years, the money poured into the March of Dimes. It paid for everything at the centers: the professional staff, patient care, equipment, and research. Later it paid for home care, home modifications, and the salaries of attendants.

Although the age incidence of polio had been rising and it was more severe in the older age groups, adults with "infantile paralysis" were treated where other childhood diseases had always been treated—the contagious wards. There, of course, the medical directors were pediatricians, so they became the medical directors of the respirator wards.

The evolution from "contagious ward" to respiratory and rehabilitation center was effected rapidly and naturally through an open-minded, learning, team approach. The typical team conference included medical director, nurse, physical therapist, occupational therapist, engineer, vocational counselor, teacher, dietitian, volunteers, and of course the patient and family.

I'm sure you all noticed that there were no pulmonologists, or respiratory therapists, on the staff. Nor was there an intensive care unit.

Regular center staff and national conferences resulted in agreement on total patient-care objectives and a consistent attitude toward the patient and family, who were seen as important members of the team.

Underlying the centers' concept of comprehensive care was the recognition of the patient as a whole human being and the perception that physical, mental, emotional, spiritual, social, and vocational problems were all interrelated. But, though their respiratory rehabilitation was successful, few patients went home until a home care plan was developed in 1953. The plan was created at Rancho Los Amigos Hospital in Los Angeles, California, to save money after a study for Los Angeles County showed that the 158 quadriplegic polio patients using respirator equipment were unnecessarily occupying hospital beds when they could be cared for at home for one-fourth the cost with attendants and supportive service.

Basically, the plan called for independence with an umbilical cord to the center. The patient remained a patient of the hospital and the patient's personal physician was placed on a Polio Physician's Panel which made the hospital staff available for consultation.

Before a patient could go home, homes were made accessible and auto-start generators were installed. Preparation for going home was extended and careful. Day long, then overnight, then weekend trial visits were made. Maintenance and service of all respiratory equipment was provided once a month and a repair truck, large enough for a lung or rocking bed, made the rounds.

In all the careful planning and adaptations there was never any attempt to move the hospital to the home and the family was involved in all planning. The family member returned home to the family—with some bulky equipment. Everyone in the family was responsible for and at ease with the equipment. They all learned to help transfer it to battery operation in a car or station wagon for trips to work or school or travel. They learned to repair and adapt it. The attitude was one of "casual carefulness."

Children were also very much a part of the home care team. A three-year old was the best aspirator I've known. She stopped the rocking bed with the foot lowered, climbed up, then, hanging upside down like a monkey, turned the bed back on. She operated the suction tubing like an orchestra conductor until she located the plug of mucus. I asked her how she did it. She said, "I watch my mommy's eyes."

At first, attendants were trained by the center. But the turnover was so rapid that it was obvious that the most effective method was to train the patient to hire and train his/her own attendants, and to train the patient to direct the operation and maintenance of ventilators.

The Rancho home care plan spread rapidly across the country and, by 1956, 92 percent of those permanently dependent upon artificial respiration equipment had been discharged to their homes.

The centers and home care resulted in tremendous financial savings and a greater degree of independence and self-sufficiency than was ever dreamed possible for people so severely disabled.

Here are a few of the cost-effective figures: the average hospital time was cut from more than a year to seven months. The home care costs were one-tenth to one-fourth of hospital costs. (Compare those costs to 1980s costs: The American Association of Respiratory Therapy 1983 survey estimated it cost $271,000 a year to maintain a ventilator-assisted person in a hospital and $21,000 at home.) Without those centers, 40 percent of those who were at home would have had to remain in custodial care for the rest of their lives.

But no figures, no statistics can measure the magic of the sharing, mutual support, caring, learning, and teaching of each other that existed between patients, families, and center staff. That learning and sharing was very evident in the gradual evolution of respiratory equipment.

In the mid-1950s, I watched the first rocking bed roll down the hall and the excitement of staff and patients over the freedom from the lung.

Next came a parade of various types and shapes of chestpieces—to fit children, a giant basketball player, and—to fit a bride—one in a special shade of pink for a wedding.

Late in the 1950s, oral positive pressure by mouthpiece was discovered. At first, it was not humidified and there were many dry mouths. Then water was added and they looked like they were smoking hubble-bubble pipes.

Just in time for a big outdoor spring picnic, the engineer at our center developed a wheelchair tray for batteries and the respirator motor. That was the forerunner for travelling ventilator users who now circle the globe.

But the Utopia of the centers and their home care programs came to an end in the late 1950s. Then the centers were closed and attendant care funds were stopped. The centers had not had permanent funding from state or federal government, but only from a voluntary agency dependent upon public largesse. When the vaccines stopped polio, the public stopped giving.

That precipitous cessation of attendant care funding in 1959 was the "burr under the saddle" that resulted in significant developments in the growth of the disability movement.

In California, the ex-patients and medical directors for the two centers effected state legislation in 1960 that created an attendant care program that is still functioning and which has grown to a multi-million dollar a year home care program for both old and young disabled persons and which has saved the state countless millions of dollars that would have been spent on institutional care.

That legislation and the successful experiences with independent living by respiratory polio survivors were the foundation for the independent living movement that was started in the 1970s in Berkeley, California, and has evolved into the disability rights movement.

In 1979, increasing problems of polio survivors with underventilation helped focus national attention on what has come to be known as the late effects of polio. Many rocking bed users and chest shell users found that they were being inadequately ventilated and they gradually switched to intermittent mouth positive pressure during the day or continuous positive airway pressure (CPAP) and face or nasal masks for night ventilation.

The large number of polio survivors experiencing problems and the need to educate other survivors and medical professionals about those problems were the catalyst for the first international polio and independent living conference in 1981 in Chicago. That first conference brought together physicians and polio survivors, several of whom travelled from as far away as Australia with their ventilators to attend.

The conferences became a biennial event, with each successive conference drawing more and more people, and more ventilator users. At the 1987 and 1989 meetings, there were special sessions on face masks with demonstrations by ventilator users of the mask systems they had designed themselves.

The application and success of home care and mechanical ventilation with respiratory polio survivors is today being transferred to individuals with high spinal cord injury, muscular dystrophy, ALS, cystic fibrosis, and, perhaps the fastest growing population, infants and young children with a variety of disabling diseases and conditions that make mechanical ventilation a necessity.

However, a few caveats:

Beware of bringing the hospital into the home.

Beware of astronomical costs involved with ventilation or society will choose the more economical alternative: no ventilators.

Beware of underestimating the limitless potential of individuals with disability.

Independence for a ventilator user means that one can say, "So *I* use a ventilator, *I* am in charge of it. *I* direct my own life and take my own risks. *I* am the one who decides about *my* quality of life."

23

PROLONGATION OF LIFE SPANS OF DUCHENNE'S MUSCULAR DYSTROPHY PATIENTS IN THE HOSPITAL CARE PROGRAM IN JAPAN

Masakuni Mukoyama, M.D.

INTRODUCTION

Patients with Duchenne's muscular dystrophy (DMD) usually die in late adolescence, but statistical data on their life spans are scarce (Emery and Skinner, 1976; Walton and Nattrass, 1954). In 1976 the Japanese Ministry of Health and Welfare established a national program which provides lifelong institutionalized care, rehabilitation, and schooling to young patients with various muscle diseases, without charge. At present, a total of 27 national sanatoria have special wards with a total of 2,500 beds for this program. Of an estimated total of 2,400 patients of DMD that survive in Japan, about half are currently hospitalized under this program (Kondo, 1980). It is our impression that the program is useful in providing high quality care, but to date, there is no information available on whether such efforts actually prolonged the life spans of the patients. In this study, we compared the life spans of DMD patients who were hospitalized under the national program with their 37 affected maternal uncles who had died at home before the introduction of the program, representing the natural course of the disease.

MATERIALS AND METHODS

Patients in this series are the 176 fatal cases with DMD who died in the wards in the period from 1970 to 1984, and for whom adequate records are available. Diagnosis was based on clinical observation for several years until the patient's death, involving repeated EMG and serum enzyme studies. Muscle biopsy was not routinely done, but was carried out in many of the cases. Atypical cases were excluded. The Becker type and so-called Fukuyama-type congenital muscular dystrophy were not included.

A collaborative research group was organized in 1978 to register fatal cases of DMD who died in these wards. Detailed case reports were collected which included agonal courses and pathological data, along with antemortem information. The present materials, therefore, were considered to represent random autopsies of unquestionable DMD cases which were admitted to these wards.

Ages at death of those who died during 1970-1974 were compared with the data of those who died during 1980-1984, and 37 affected maternal uncles.

RESULTS

All patients were males. The age of death of the 176 patients ranged from 10 to 29 years, with a mode at 18 and a mean of 18.28 ± 3.55 years. The curve was unimodal. The age of death in 48 patients who died between 1980 and 1984 ranged from 14 to 28 and averaged 19.96 ± 3.90 years, whereas 63 patients who died between 1970 and 1974 ranged from 10 to 29 and averaged 17.81 ± 3.68 years. The former group lived significantly longer than the latter ($p < 0.005$).

Thirty-seven affected maternal uncles had a life span of 5 to 30 years, with an average of 17.24 ± 4.69 years. This was lower than that of the total 176 patients ($0.05 < p < 0.1$), and was significantly lower than that of the recently hospitalized group that died between 1980 and 1984 ($p < 0.005$).

Pulmonary infection was the most frequent cause of demise in the group of patients who died from1970 to 1974 than in those who died between 1980 and 1984 (25.4 percent vs. 8.3 percent). Respiratory insufficiency as a cause of death was more common in the latter group (37.5 percent vs. 9.5 percent).

DISCUSSION

The study indicated that 1) hospitalized patients had longer average life spans than their affected uncles, who died without proper care before the national program was set up; 2) patients hospitalized recently lived longer than those hospitalized in the past, soon after the introduction of the program; and 3) while pulmonary infection has become a less frequent cause of death, respiratory insufficiency is a more common cause of death in current cases. These changes have occurred in correlation with severe dystrophic alterations of the diaphragm and intercostal muscles, which were observed at autopsy (Mukoyama, et al., 1984). The data summarize reports by pathologists from the different institutes at the different dates. Pathological descriptions were somewhat arbitrary, but we believe that they indicated a shift in the cause of death in DMD patients over the last decade and reflected the benefits of the program, in which complications, especially infections, were maximally eliminated, and dystrophic changes more directly caused the death of patients.

It is likely that recent prolongation of life is due to better management: controlled nutrition, prevention and treatment of cardiopulmonary complications (Matsuo, 1983; Mukoyama and Kohno, 1979), and utilization of ventilators (Curran and Colbert, 1989). Various social and psychological issues have been raised recently in Japan about DMD patients on long-term ventilator life-support.

SUMMARY

Analysis of the results of the 176 autopsies of DMD patients demonstrated that 1) hospitalized patients had longer life spans than their non-hospitalized affected maternal uncles; 2) patients hospitalized recently lived longer than those hospitalized in the past; and 3) pulmonary infection has become a less frequent cause of death, whereas dystrophic changes of the cardiac and respiratory muscles are more closely related with more recent fatal cases. The results indicate a changing life span expectancy of patients with DMD and changes in cause of death over the last decade, probably owing to the benefits of a hospital care program.

REFERENCES

Curran, F.J., and A.P. Colbert, "Ventilator Management in Duchenne Muscular Dystrophy and Postpoliomyelitis Syndrome: Twelve Years Experience," *Arch Phys Med Rehabil*, 1989, 70: 180–185.

Emery, A.E.H., and R. Skinner, "Clinical Studies in Benign (Becker type) X-linked Muscular Dystrophy," *Clin Genet*, 1976, 10:189–201.

Kondo, K., "Genetics of Duchenne Muscular Dystrophy and Care Program in Japan," *Adv Neurol Sci* (Tokyo), 1980, 24: 693–701.

Matsuo, S., "Respiratory Failure and Its Prevention in Duchenne Muscular Dystrophy," *IRYO* (Official publication of the national hospitals and sanatoria of Japan), 1983, 37: 474–481.

Mukoyama, M., K. Hizawa, K. Hayashi, and I. Sobue, "The Life Span, Causes of Death and Pathological Findings of Duchenne Muscular Dystrophy: Analysis of 124 Autopsy Cases," *Neurol Med* (Tokyo), 1984, 20: 377–380.

Mukoyama, M., and K. Kohno, "Pathology of the Heart in Duchenne Type Muscular Dystrophy. Comparison with ECG Findings," *Abstract 2nd International Child Neurology Congress*, 1979, p.158.

Walton, J.N., and F.J. Nattrass, "On the Classification, Natural History and Treatment of Myopathies," *Brain*, 1954, 77: 169–231.

24

CARDIOVASCULAR ABNORMALITIES IN DUCHENNE'S MUSCULAR DYSTROPHY

Radha J. Sarma, M.B.B.S., F.A.C.C., F.A.C.P.
Syed Ejaz Naqvi, M.B.B.S.
Sekhar C. Kota, M.B.B.S.
Robert Sudrann, M.D.

INTRODUCTION

Duchenne's muscular dystrophy (DMD) is a progressive, sex-linked recessive disorder that affects the skeletal muscles and the heart. There are several cardiac abnormalities in DMD, none of which are either specific or pathognomonic for this condition alone. Death before the age of 20 has been reported in the past (Gardner-Medwin, 1980). Gilroy (1963) reported that death was related to respiratory insufficiency in most of the patients but cardiac failure was the second most common cause in these patients. Becker in 1955 described a slowly progressive muscular dystrophy that is considered a distinct entity from DMD; these patients are ambulatory until they are older. The cardiovascular abnormalities are similar to those in DMD. Recent advances in mechanical ventilation have raised hopes of prolonging longevity in this group of patients (Curran, 1981; Rideau, 1983) and now cardiomyopathy is increasingly recognized as an important cause of mortality and morbidity. Hence, the diagnosis and treatment of cardiac abnormalities are important aspects of the total care of DMD patients.

DETECTION OF CARDIAC INVOLVEMENT

History and Symptoms

Patients may complain of palpitations and dyspnea; in ventilator-dependent patients the dyspnea may not be accurately identified as due to cardiac failure. In patients with respiratory infections, symptoms of heart failure may be misinterpreted. Two cases were described in the literature (Seay, 1978), with cardiac arrest during anesthesia as the initial presentation of DMD cardiac involvement. Another case, of a 19-year-old male who presented in acute pulmonary edema without a prior diagnosis of muscular dystrophy, was described by Borgeat (1987). This suggests that clinicians should be aware of the common as well as the unusual cardiac presentations of muscular dystrophy.

Physical Examination

There may be no abnormal findings on physical examination of the heart in some patients. In others with striking thoracic deformities, there may be abnormal heart sounds and murmurs. Perloff (1966) described the presence of a soft midsystolic murmur in the second left intercostal space, loud pulmonic component of the second heart sound, although it is not usually due to pulmonary hypertension. Murmur of mitral regurgitation is usually secondary to mitral valve prolapse. When congestive heart failure occurs, presence of third heart sound, jugular venous distension and, rarely, pulmonary rales may be detected. In patients confined to bed, edema of the extremities is not usually seen.

Diagnostic Testing

Until recently, the electrocardiogram, vectorcardiogram, and chest x-ray were the routine tests used for diagnosing cardiac abnormalities. With the availability of nuclear cardiologic testing and echocardiography, it is now possible to detect minor abnormalities in cardiac anatomy and function more easily and more accurately. The usefulness and limitations of the tests are as follows:

Electrocardiogram (ECG)

The typical electrocardiogram in DMD is one with tall R wave and in ratio over 1 in the right precordial leads (Perloff, 1967; Weisenfeld, 1952). Sanyal in 1978 reported this pattern in 64 percent of their 75 patients; in 44 percent of the patients, they noted Q waves < 4 mm deep in lead 1, aVL, and or V5 and V6 mimicking anterolateral myocardial infarction. Two other types were described by Slucka in 1968; one where the V1 lead shows rSr′

and the second where the r wave is polyphasic. The EKG may also be normal at times.

A short PR interval without delta waves was found in up to 50 percent of patients (Perloff, 1984). Although intracardiac electrophysiological studies are not available in DMD, the short PR interval may represent atrio-fascicular bypass tract or accelerated conduction within the AV node. At our institution we are following a patient who had a short PR interval at entry but later manifested the delta wave typical of the Wolf Parkinson White type of preexcitation. Other less common ECG findings include right axis deviation and left axis deviation.

ECG is the simplest and most reliable tool for detecting cardiac involvement in DMD. Abnormal ECGs are present even in early childhood (Slucka, 1968). Lane (1980) suggested that the typical ECG pattern is also helpful in detecting carrier women and confirmed earlier findings by Emery (1969). They found that the sum of R-S amplitude in lead V1 and the R/S ratio in leads V1 and V2 was significantly greater in carrier females than in age-matched controls.

The tall R waves and deep Q waves described above are considered to be secondary to reduction in or a loss of electrical activity caused by dystrophic changes in the posterobasal left ventricular wall and the contiguous lateral wall, respectively (Perloff, 1967; Sanyal, 1978). Sequential changes such as the high frequency notches in QRS complexes have been reported to be useful indicators for estimating the extent and severity of cardiac involvement (Ishikawa, 1979).

However, the prognostic value of the EKG is not very good, as there is no significant correlation between clinical course and either the degree of ECG abnormality or the level of cardiac enzymes (Slucka, 1968).

High frequency signal averaged EKG (late potentials). Our experience at Rancho Los Amigos Medical center in 25 DMD patients showed a trend toward increased incidence of late potentials and ventricular arrhythmias in patients with markedly decreased left ventricular ejection fraction (LVEF). However, more data is needed to draw firm conclusions in DMD patients, as the nature of the disease process is different from the usual coronary artery disease patients with myocardial infarctions.

Arrhythmias and conduction defects. In the presence of severe chest deformities and respirators, some times it may be difficult to obtain good quality 24-hour Holter monitor studies in DMD patients. Southall and others in 1981 described 24-hour Holter findings in 104 randomly selected healthy children between 7 and 11 years of age. The results of the study may give some idea of the frequency of minor common arrhythmias occurring in normal healthy children. Surprisingly, many DMD patients also show similar arrhythmias. Conduction defects can occur anywhere between the sinus node to the His-Purkinji system. Perloff (1984) described abnormal intraatrial or interatrial conduction, Mobitz type 1 block, nonconducted atrial premature beats, short P-R interval, right ventricular conduction delay and right axis deviation suggestive of left posterior fascicular block in 20 patients with DMD. Sanyal (1978) found widely scattered focal dystrophic changes in the heart, involving atrial and ventricular myocardium, ventricular septum, papillary muscle, and conduction system. The dystrophic changes were similar to those of skeletal muscles in these patients. These abnormal dystrophic changes may be the cause of the conduction defects and arrhythmias seen in this group of patients. Thickening of small intramural coronary arteries as a cause of the dystrophic and fibrotic changes in the myocardium remains speculative (Perloff, 1967).

Arrhythmias. Sinus tachycardia, labile or persistent, is the most common arrhythmias. Abnormal autonomic regulation has also been implicated as a cause of sinus tachycardia (Perloff, 1984). Sinus pause, premature atrial contractions, and atrial flutter may also occur. Premature ventricular beats and ventricular tachycardia are less common. Except for end stage atrial flutter, these abnormalities are not usually clinically deleterious. Supraventricular arrhythmias generally are more common than ventricular arrhythmias. The exact mechanism of these arrhythmias is not established.

Vectorcardiograms

Fitch (1967) described Frank vector cardiograms in 44 DMD patients. Abnormalities were noted in 95 percent, and they did not have any correlation to the age of the patient or the severity of the disease. Ronan (1972) also described vector findings in their patients. It is interesting that the vector loop in the horizontal plane was never clockwise, in spite of the electrocardiographic tall R waves in anterior precordial leads; on the other hand, in right ventricular hypertrophy the horizontal loop is frequently clockwise.

Systolic time intervals (STI). STI measurements are usually obtained from simultaneous high-speed recording of ECG, carotid pulse tracing, and phonocardiogram. Echocardiograms were also used to obtain the same measurements. The value of STI measurements has become well established as a sensitive noninvasive means of evaluating global left ventricular performance. STI abnormalities are common in children with DMD (Sanyal, 1982), prolonged preejection period/left ventricular ejection time ratio being the single most useful measurement to indicate deterioration in the cardiac status, and serial studies of STI may provide means of evaluating the progression of cardiomyopathy in these patients (Hunsaker, 1982).

Echocardiography

M-mode echocardiography was used extensively in the past to detect mitral valve prolapse, calculate the posterior wall systolic and diastolic maximal velocities, left ventricular wall thickness and mass, fractional shortening (FS), and ejection fraction (EF). Because of the severe chest and spine deformities in DMD patients, echocardiograms may not always be of good quality, and the routine measurements may not be accurate.

Two-dimensional echocardiogram (2DE) is more useful than M-modo examination alone. 2DE is most useful in the detection of mitral valve prolapse (MVP), regional wall motion abnormalities, and measurement of FS and EF. Serial measurements of FS and EF serve as useful guides to follow progression of cardiomyopathy and also to evaluate response to therapy. The addition of color flow mapping and Doppler methods to M-mode and 2DE makes it easier to detect regurgitation across the valves and calculate intracardiac hemodynamics. Systolic and diasolic velocity measurements, however, are calculated more accurately using high speed recordings from the M-mode echocardiograms. Abnormalities detected by echocardiography in DMD patients are as follows:

Mitral valve prolapse (MVP). MVP occurs frequently in patients with DMD. Reported incidence varies from 11 percent (Danilowicz, 1980) to 55 percent (Sanyal, 1979). Reeves, et al. (1980) reported MVP in 25 percent of their 24 patients. One of the reasons for this wide range may be the different echocardiographic criteria used by different investigators. The majority of these patients have systolic click (early, mid, or late) on physical exam. Biddison, et al. (1979) found a higher incidence of MVP in families with x-linked muscular dystrophy (DMD or Becker type) including the carrier mothers. The cause of MVP is widely believed to be secondary to thoracic deformities or dystrophic involvement of the papillary muscle and ventricular myocardium (Sanyal, 1980). Mitral valve leaflets, annulus, or chordae tendinae themselves are usually normal, although Biddison, et al. (1979) found myxomatous degeneration of mitral valve leaflets in two patients with MVP. Reeves, et al. (1980), in their series, found skeletal muscle deformities in all patients with MVP and DMD, but none with myotonic muscular dystrophy and MVP. It is important to note that Perloff (1984) reported that MVP is rarely a cause of rhythm disturbance in these patients. Generally no antibiotic prophylaxis is necessary unless there is associated mitral regurgitation.

Left ventricular posterior wall. Decrease in maximal systolic and diastolic endocardial velocity is a typical diagnostic finding in this condition (Ahmad, 1977; Farah, 1980; Goldberg, 1980; Kovick, 1973). Decreased wall thickness in DMD patients as compared to age-matched controls has been reported by Goldberg (1983).

Left ventricular size and function. Dilatation of the left ventricle with increased mass, as well as atrophic left ventricle with decreased mass, may occur in these patients. Abnormal wall motion may be noted initially in the posterior wall only and may extend to the inferior wall, anterior wall, lateral wall, apex, and to the septum in later stages (Goldberg, 1982). FS and EF may be decreased in the advanced cases (Heymsfield, 1978; Ishikawa, 1981). At our institution, one 17-year-old black male with Becker's muscular dystrophy had a dilated, poorly contracting left ventricle with a large mural thrombus at the left ventricular apex; several others had severely depressed left ventricular ejection fraction. We did not find good correlation between the age of the patient, the degree of skeletal muscle involvement, and the poor left ventricular function. Others reported findings suggesting the correlation in some (Hunsaker, 1982), and no correlation (Farah, 1980) in others.

Other cardiac chambers. Left atrial enlargement may be seen when the mitral regurgitation is moderate to severe or when the left ventricle is dilated and the EF is decreased. Towards the later stages of cardiomyopathy with congestive heart failure, the right ventricle and right atrium may show volume overload and tricuspid regurgitation.

Radionuclide Studies

One of the most commonly used and fairly reliable tests is the gated radionuclide ventriculogram (RNV or MUGA). From this test it is possible to detect wall motion abnormalities and measure EF. Other less commonly used tests are Thallium-201 myocardial perfusion scan, Technicium Pyrophosphate scan, and positron emission computed tomography (PET scan) to study the regional myocardial metabolism. These tests are useful in following the progression of cardiomyopathy in DMD patients.

Radionuclide ventriculography. At our institution, Stewart and Gilgoff (1988) reported the usefulness of RNV to estimate EF in DMD patients and the prognostic value of markedly decreased EF in predicting mortality. Iorio, et al. (1988) reported that equilibrium RNV performed at rest and after hand grip exercise in 20 DMD patients showed generally a reduction in EF and an increase in wall motion abnormalities. Stewart and others at our institution are currently conducting gated RNV and Thallium 201 studies using transesophageal pacing; one patient showed decrease in the EF, while others showed an increase in EF. This may be an easy way to determine the cardiac reserve in these patients, although experience with a large number of patients is necessary to prove the usefulness of this technique.

Thallium 201 myocardial perfusion imaging. Perloff, et al. (1984) performed RNV, Thallium-201 perfusion imaging, PET imaging echocardiograms, and electrocardiograms in 20 DMD patients, to evaluate the metabolic abnormalities in areas of the heart known to be affected by the dystrophic process at necropsy. They found increased exogenous glucose utilization in the posterobasal wall using F-18 deoxy glucose with PET scanning, and in the same regions 13NH3 activity was decreased, suggesting either a regional metabolic alteration in uptake and trapping, a decrease in regional blood flow, or both. Nagamachi, et al. (1989) found Thallium-201 perfusion defects in the absence of coronary artery disease in DMD patients. It is postulated that regional reduction in myocardial blood flow is related to a decrease in muscle fiber content per unit mass (fibrous replacement). Most of these areas are present in posterior and inferior walls and tend to become more prominent with age and severity of the disease process. Yamamoto (1988) reported that Thallium perfusion defects in the posterobasal area of the left ventricle are frequent in DMD patients, along with EKG abnormalities. However, they concluded that in the total population of the muscular dystrophies the ECG may be underestimating the degree of fibrosis. In addition to the Thallium defects, the other interesting abnormalities detected in this study are malrotation, apical aneurysms, and dilatation of the left ventricle. The prognostic value of Thallium imaging is worth mentioning. Kawai (1985) reported that two patients with extensive Thallium defects died of congestive heart failure within two years of the study. In their study, the progression of the defects was considered minimal over a two- to three-year period. Jinnouchi (1985) reported extension of Thallium defects with age and stage. However, Nagamachi (1989) reported the progression of Thallium defects in DMD patients who were studied by serial Thallium imaging over a period of two years.

Pyrophosphate heart scintigrams. Duska (1984) reported the results of Pyrophosphate scintigraphy in 16 boys with advanced DMD as indicated by their EKG and enzyme values. Abnormal results were noted in 7 of the 16 patients; in 4 patients they were clearly positive and, in 3, borderline. There was no correlation between the duration of the disease or the degree of skeletal muscle involvement and the abnormalities on the scintigrams. There was a general positive correlation between the enzyme level and the abnormal scintigrams. As pyrophosphate scans detect recent progression of myocardial cell damage, the abnormalities indicate recent events, but already damaged and fibrosed areas may not be picked up by this test. Interestingly, the affected skeletal muscles in the patients with abnormal scintigrams did not show any increased uptake of the isotope. This may suggest the disease progression in the heart and the muscles is not concurrent in this group.

Pathology of Cardiomyopathy in DMD

The early cardiac involvement in DMD is characterized by fibrosis of the epicardial half of the posterior base of the left ventricle. The interventricular septum rarely shows fibrosis. The fibrosis is not similar to that observed in myocardial infarction; in DMD, normal myocardial cells are intermixed with fibrotic areas (Frankel and Rosser, 1976). In this report, only two of the eight patients had a heart weight under 200 gms, while in the other six the heart weight ranged from 250 to 450 gms. Right ventricular involvement in the dystrophic process was rare. The valves have been described to be normal in the report by Frankel and Rosser (1976), although myxomatous degeneration of the mitral valve was described by Biddison (1979). Abnormalities involving the cardiac conduction system and the small coronary arteries were described by James (1962).

TREATMENT OF CARDIAC COMPLICATIONS IN DMD

Ideally, treatment should be aimed at the cellular dystrophic process, to prevent either metabolic or structural abnormalities. So far, several attempts have been made to treat the skeletal muscle weakness by using a variety of drugs and physical therapy. These studies did not evaluate the cardiac improvement. One study reported beneficial results in treating the cardiac involvement by using the coenzyme Q10 (Folkers, 1985), but the agent is not easily available for clinical use. Still,there is no specific therapy for the cardiac disease in DMD. Most of the treatment aspects are mainly aimed at preventing death due to congestive heart failure or arrhythmias. Digitalis and diuretics have been found to be effective in a few reports (Mattioli and Melhorn, 1982). At our institution over the past two years, we find the use of angiotensin converting enzyme inhibitors very useful in treating adult muscular dystrophy patients with poor left ventricular ejection fraction and congestive heart failure. Further research in this area is important to prevent cardiac mortality and morbidity in DMD patients.

REFERENCES

Ahmad, M., J.E. Sanderson, V. Dubowitz, and K.A. Hallidie-Smith, "Echocardiographic Assessment of Left Ventricular Function in Duchenne's Muscular Dystrophy," *British Heart Journal* 1978, 40: 734–740.

Becker, P.E., and F. Keiner, "Eine neue x-chromosomale Muskeldystrophie," *Archiv fur Psychiatrie und Nervenkrankheiten vereinigt mit Zeitschrift fur die gesamte Neurologie und Psychiatrie* 1955, 193: 427–448.

Biddison, J.H., D.H. Dembo, H. Spalt, M.G. Hayes, and C.W. LeDoux, "Familial Occurrence of Mitral Valve Prolapse in X-linked Muscular Dystrophy," *Circulation* 1979, 59: 1299–1304.

Borgeat, A., J.J. Goy, and U. Sigwart, "Acute Pulmonary Edema as the Inaugural Symptom of Becker's Muscular Dystrophy in a 19-Year Old Patient," *Clinical Cardiology* 1987, 10: 127-129.

Danilowicz, D., M. Rutlowski, D. Myung, and D. Schively, "Echocardiography in Duchenne Muscular Dystrophy," *Muscle and Nerve* 1980, 3: 298–303.

Duska, F., Z. Nesvadba, P. Zdansky, J. Novak, J. Kubicek, P. Kafka, J. Vizda, and Mazurova, "The Pyrophosphate Heart Scintigram in Children With Progressive Muscular Dystrophy," *Nuclear Medicine* 1984, 23: 189–191.

Emery, A.E.H., "Abnormalities of the Electrocardiogram in Female Carriers of Duchenne Muscular Dystrophy," *British Medical Journal* 1969, 2:418–420.

Farah, M.C., E.B. Evans, and P.J. Vignos, "Echocardiographic Evaluation of Left Ventricular Function in Duchenne's Muscular Dystrophy," *American Journal of Medicine* 1980, 69: 248–254.

Fitch, C.W., and L.W. Ainger, "The Frank Vectorcardiogram and the Electrocardiogram in Duchenne Progressive Muscular Dystrophy," *Circulation* 1967, 35: 1124–1140.

Folkers, K., J. Wolaniuk, and R. Simonsen, et al., "Biochemical Rationale and the Cardiac Response of Patients With Muscle Disease to Therapy With Coenzyme Q10," *Proceedings of the National Academy of Sciences* 1985, 82: 4513–4516.

Frankel, K.A., and R.J. Rosser, "The Pathology of the Heart in Progressive Muscular Dystrophy: Epimyocardial Fibrosis," *Human Pathology* 1976, 7: 375–386.

Gardner-Medwin, D., "Clinical Features and Classification of the Muscular Dystrophies," *British Medical Bulletin* 1980, 36 No 2: 109–115.

Gilroy, J., J.L. Cahalan, R. Berman, and M. Newman, "Cardiac and Pulmonary Complications in Duchenne's Progressive Muscular Dystrophy," *Circulation* 1963, 27: 484–493.

Goldberg, S.J., L. Feldman, C. Reinecke, L.Z. Stern, D. Sahn, and H.D. Allen, "Echocardiographic Determination of Contraction and Relaxation Measurements of the Left Ventricular Wall in Normal Subjects and Patients With Muscular Dystrophy," *Circulation* 1980, 62: 1061–1069.

Goldberg, S.J., L.Z. Stern, L. Feldman, H.D. Allen, D. Sahn, and L.M. Valdes-Cruz, "Serial Two-dimensional Echocardiography in Duchenne Muscular Dystrophy," *Neurology* 1982, 32: 1101–1105.

Goldberg, S.J., L.Z. Stern, L. Feldman, D. Sahn, H.D. Allen, and L.M. Valdes-Cruz, "Serial Left Ventricular Wall Measurements in Duchenne's

Muscular Dystrophy," *Journal of the American College of Cardiology* 1983, 2: 136–142.

Heymsfield, S.B., T. McNish, J.V. Perkins, and J.M. Felner, "Sequence of Cardiac Changes in Duchenne Muscular Dystrophy," *American Heart Journal* 1978, 95: 283–294.

Hunsaker, R.H., P.K. Fulkerson, F.J. Barry, R.P. Lewis, C.V. Leier, and D.V. Unverferth, "Cardiac Function in Duchenne's Muscular Dystrophy. Results of 10 Year Follow-up Study and Noninvasive Test," *American Journal of Medicine* 1982, 73: 235–238.

Iorio, F., L.M. Ferro, I. Genvini, F. Scopinaro, and C.A. Centi, "Equilibrium Radionuclide Ventriculography in Duchenne's Cardiomyopathy," *Nuclear Medicine Communication* 1988, 9: 357–61.

Ishikawa, K., H. Kanemitsu, T. Ishihara, T. Tamura, H. Shimada, and M. Inoue, "Echocardiographic Study of the Duchenne Type of Progressive Muscular Dystrophy," *Japanese Circulation Journal* 1981, 45: 295–301.

Ishikawa, K., A. Yanagisawa, T. Ishihara, T. Tamura, and M. Inoue, "Sequential Changes of Orthogonal Electrocardiograms in Progressive Muscular Dystrophy of the Duchenne Type," *American Heart Journal* 1979, 98: 73–82.

James, T.N., "Observations on the Cardiovascular Involvement, Including the Cardiac Conduction System, in Progressive Muscular Dystrophy," *American Heart Journal* 1962, 63: 48–56.

Jinnouchi, S., J. Asai, K. Inoue, H. Hoshi, and K. Watanabe, "Evaluation of Cardiomyopathy in Duchenne Muscular Dystrophy by TI-201 Myocardial SPECT," *Japanese Journal of Nuclear Medicine* 1985, 22: 1353–1359.

Kawai, N., I. Sotobata, M. Okada, M. Iwase, S. Yamamoto, H. Matsushima, H. Miyakoda, M. Yokota, K. Yamauchi, and Hayashi, "Evaluation of Myocardial Involvement in Duchenne Progressive Muscular Dystrophy With Thallium-201 Myocardial Perfusion Imaging," *Japanese Heart Journal* 1985, 5: 767–775.

Kovick, R.B., A.M. Fogelman, A.S. Abbasi, J.B. Peter, and M.I. Pearce, "Echocardiographic Evaluation of Posterior Left Ventricular Wall Motion in Muscular Dystrophy," *Circulation* 1975, 52: 447–454.

Lane, R.J.M., D. Gardner-Medwin, and A.D. Roses, "Electrocardiographic Abnormalities in Carriers of Duchenne Muscular Dystrophy," *Neurology* 1980, 30: 497–501.

Mattioli, L., and M. Melhorn, "Duchenne's Muscular Dystrophy," *The Journal of Kansas Medical Society* 1982, 115–121.

Nagamachi, S., S. Jinnouchi, S. Ono, H. Hoshi, K. Inoue, and K. Watanabe, "TI-201 Myocardial SPECT in Patients With Duchenne's Muscular Dystrophy: A Long Term Follow Up," *Clinical Nuclear Medicine* 1989, 14: 827–830.

Perloff, J.K., "Cardiac Rhythm and Conduction in Duchenne's Muscular Dystrophy: A Prospective Study of 20 Patients," *Journal of the American College of Cardiology* 1984, 3: 1263–1268.

Perloff, J.K., A.C. De Leon, and D. O'Doherty, "The Cardiomyopathy of Progressive Muscular Dystrophy," *Circulation* 1966, 33: 625–648.

Perloff, J.K., E. Henze, and H. Schelbert, "Alterations in Regional Myocardial Metabolism, Perfusion, and Wall Motion in Duchenne Muscular Dystrophy Studied by Radionuclide Imaging," *Circulation* 1984, 69: 33–42.

Perloff, J.K., W.C. Roberts, A.C. DeLeon, and O'Doherty, "The Distinctive Electrocardiogram of Duchenne's Progressive Muscular Dystrophy: An Electrocardiographic-Pathologic Correlative Study," *American Journal of Medicine* 1967, 42: 179–188.

Reeves, W.C., R. Griggs, N.C. Nanda, K. Thomson, and R. Gramiak, "Echocardiographic Evaluation of Cardiac Abnormalities in Duchenne's Dystrophy and Myotonic Muscular Dystrophy," *Archives of Neurology* 1980, 37: 273–277.

Rideau, Y., G. Gatin, J. Bach, and G. Gines, "Prolongation of Life in Duchennes's Muscular Dystrophy," *Acta Neurology* 1983, 5: 118–124.

Ronan, J.A., J.K. Perloff, P.J. Bowen, and O. Mann, "The Vectorcardiogram in Duchenne's Progressive Muscular Dystrophy," *American Heart Journal* 1972, 84: 588–596.

Sanyal, S.K., W.W. Johnson, M.R. Dische, S. Pitner, and C. Beard, "Dystrophic Degeneration of Papillary Muscle and Ventricular Myocardium," *Circulation* 1980, 62: 430–437.

Sanyal, S.K., W.W. Johnson, M.K. Thapar, and S. Pitner, "An Ultrastructural Basis for Electrocardiographic Alterations Associated With Duchenne's Progressive Muscular Dystrophy," *Circulation* 1978, 57: 1122–1129.

Sanyal, S.K., R.K.F. Leung, R.C. Tierney, R. Gillmartin, and S. Pitner, "Mitral Valve Prolapse Syndrome in Children With Duchenne's Progressive Muscular Dystrophy," *Pediatrics* 1979, 63: 116–122.

Sanyal, S.K., R.C. Tierney, Rao P. Syamasunder, S. Pitner, S.L. George, and D. Givins, "Systolic Time Interval Characteristics in Children With Duchenne's Progressive Muscular Dystrophy," *Pediatrics* 1982, 70: 958–954.

Seay, A.R., F. Ziter, and J.A. Thompson, "Cardiac Arrest During Anesthesia in Duchenne Muscular Dystrophy," *The Journal of Pediatrics* 1978, 93: 88-90.

Slucka, C., "The Electrocardiogram in Duchenne Progressive Muscular Dystrophy," *Circulation* 1968, 38: 933–940.

Southall, D.P., F. Johnston, E.A. Shinebourne, and P.G.B. Johnston, "24-hour Electrocardiographic Study of Heart Rate and Rhythm Patterns in Population of Healthy Children," *British Heart Journal* 1981, 45: 281–291.

Stewart, C.A., I. Gilgoff, A. Baydur, and W. Prentice, "Gated Radionuclide Ventriculography in the Evaluation of Cardiac Function in Duchenne's Muscular Dystrophy," *Chest* 1988, 94: 1245–1248.

Weisenfeld, A., and W.J. Messinger, "Cardiac Involvement in Progressive Muscular Dystrophy," *American Heart Journal* 1952, 43: 170–187.

Yamamoto, S., H. Matsushima, A. Suzuki, I. Sotobata, and T. Indo, et al., "A Comparative Study of Thallium-201 Single-photon Emission Computed Tomography and Electrocardiography in Duchenne and Other Types of Muscular Dystrophy," *The American Journal of Cardiology* 1988, 61: 836–843.

APPENDIX

The following are the legends for figures from two interesting cases.

CASE 1

A 17-year-old black male with Becker's Muscular Dystrophy. Not on a respirator and is ambulating.

EKG showing typical tall R waves in right pericardial leads and deep Q waves in lateral pericardial leads.

M-mode echocardiogram at the mitral valve level showing mitral valve prolapse.

Two-dimensional echocardiogram (top) showing the cursor where the M-mode echocardiogram (bottom) was obtained. The left ventricle is dilated with poor contraction of the posterior wall and septum.

CASE 2

A 44-year-old white male with Duchenne's Muscular Dystrophy on a ventilator in wheelchair.

EKG on 9/27/88 shows typical W-P-W type pre-excitation with delta waves.

EKG on 4/5/89 shows supraventricular tachycardia with left axis deviation.

25

A HISTORICAL PERSPECTIVE ON THE USE OF NONINVASIVE VENTILATORY SUPPORT ALTERNATIVES

John R. Bach, M.D.

And the Lord God formed man of the dust of the ground, and gave him positive pressure ventilation via nasal access, the breath of life.

Genesis 2:7

INTRODUCTION

Respiratory failure is the most common cause of death of patients with traumatic quadriplegia (1,2) and progressive neuromuscular disease (3). Insidiously progressive chronic ventilatory insufficiency, which not infrequently complicates post-poliomyelitis, post-spinal cord injury, obesity/hypoventilation syndrome, kyphoscoliosis, and chronic obstructive pulmonary disease, among other conditions, commonly leads to cor pulmonale, cardiopulmonary failure and death. The lives of many of these patients can be significantly prolonged by long-term ventilatory support; however, most patients refuse elective tracheostomy for intermittent positive pressure ventilation (IPPV). Likewise, electrophrenic respiration (EPR) with a phrenic nerve pacemaker has few indications and is often unsuccessful. It, too, requires surgical procedures and usually requires the long-term presence of a tracheostomy tube.

The noninvasive modalities of ventilatory support are used in relatively few centers, and few clinicians are familiar with all of the techniques available, but there has been interest of late in exploring their use as alternatives to tracheostomy IPPV. These noninvasive methods include the use of body ventilators, and the more recently described noninvasive intermittent direct positive airway pressure methods. The body ventilators include the Iron Lung, Porta-Lung, Chest Shell, wrap ventilators, and the intermittent abdominal pressure ventilator. The noninvasive intermittent positive airway pressure techniques include IPPV via the mouth, nose, and oral-nasal interfaces.

HISTORICAL PERSPECTIVE

Mechanical ventilatory support may have first been attempted by Paraceleus, who was given credit for using a chimney bellows to inflate the lungs of moribund or recently deceased individuals around 1530. This technique of using a chimney bellows to deliver IPPV through the mouth for patient resuscitation continued to be used in Europe through the nineteenth century (4).

Body Ventilators

Negative pressure body ventilators include the tank or cuirass styles. Tank ventilators consist of either a cylinder or a tank which contains the patient with only the head protruding, i.e., the Iron Lung (Emerson Co., Cambridge, MA) or Porta-Lung (Porta-Lung Inc., Denver, CO). The cuirass style ventilators consist of a firm shell which covers the chest and abdomen, i.e., the Chest Shell Ventilator (Lifecare, Inc., Lafayette, CO; Puritan-Bennett, Boulder, CO) (5). By either of these methods, negative pressure is created around parts of the body, including the thorax and the abdomen, and inspiration occurs passively to equalize the pressures inside and outside of the tank or cuirass. Negative pressure is created in the Iron Lung by the action of a bellows mechanism. Negative pressure is created under the shell of the Chest Shell or in the Porta-Lung by the action of a negative pressure pump or ventilator through a connecting hose.

The first body ventilator, a tank ventilator, was described by the Scottish physician John Dalziel in 1832 (6). Negative pressure was created by a pair of bellows operated by a piston rod. Successful use of similar devices, including the cuirass style ventilators, was described a few years later (7,8). The first body ventilator to receive widespread use, however, was the Iron Lung developed by Drinker and Shaw in 1928 (8). The Emerson Iron Lungs developed in 1931 were the main devices used prior to 1952 to provide 24-hour long-term ventilatory support and, in particular, nocturnal ventilatory support for patients with paralytic/restrictive respiratory failure. These Iron Lungs continue to be manufactured, and are used by many today.

The Rocking Bed is another style of negative pressure body ventilator that has been used since 1932 to support the ventilation of patients with poliomyelitis or muscular dystrophy (9). The Rocking Bed (Emerson Co., Cambridge, MA) rocks the patient from 15° to 30° off the horizontal and uses gravity to create cyclical displacement of the abdominal contents, which causes sufficient diaphragmatic excursion to ventilate the patient. Although the device is adequate to ventilate patients with relatively normal pulmonary mechanics, it cannot move as much air as the tank or cuirass ventilators (10). It, like the Iron Lung, continues to be manufactured and used by many (11).

Although various types of cuirass ventilators have been described since 1832 (7), the Fairchild-Huxley chest respirator (12) and the Monaghan Portable Respirator (13) were introduced in 1949 and became the first mass-produced cuirasses which covered only the anterior thorax and upper abdomen. They were reported to be used for long-term supported daytime ventilation, with the patient sitting erect, as well as for nocturnal support. Similar cuirasses or chest shells are manufactured today and are used predominately for nocturnal ventilatory assistance (Lifecare, Inc., Lafayette, CO; Puritan-Rennett, Boulder, CO). Their use for daytime aid has been largely supplanted by more practical methods, including intermittent positive airway pressure supported ventilation, the intermittent abdominal pressure ventilator, and glossopharyngeal breathing (14).

The "wrap ventilators" are the most recently developed negative pressure body ventilators. The prototype wrap ventilator was the Tunnicliffe breathing jacket, which was described in 1955 and continues to be used in England (15). It, and the wrap ventilators that followed it, work on the same principle as the Chest Shell. They consist of a firm plastic grid covering at least the anterior thorax and upper abdomen. The grid and the body under it are covered by a wind-proof jacket, which is sealed around the patient's neck and extremities. As negative pressure is cycled under the wrap and grid, air enters via the upper airway to ventilate the patient. The only significant changes in modern wrap ventilators from the original design are the materials used to fabricate the jacket and the length and form of the extremity sleeves (16). Although more time-consuming to don, wrap ventilators are more effective when carefully placed and correctly used, because of better covering of the thorax and abdomen.

Another style of body ventilator which is driven by a positive pressure ventilator or cycling pump is the intermittent abdominal pressure ventilator (Exsufflation belt, Lifecare, Inc., Lafayette, CO), or Pneumobelt (Puritan-Bennett, Inc., Boulder, CO). The prototype of this ventilator was the Bragg-Paul Pulsator, which was described by C.J. McSweeney in 1938. "The apparatus . . . consists of a distensible rubber bag applied around the patient's chest in the form of a belt, this belt being rhythmically filled with, and emptied of, air" (17). The modern abdominal pressure ventilator (18) consists of an elastic inflatable bladder incorporated within an abdominal corset worn beneath the patient's outer clothing. The bladder compresses the abdomen when cyclically inflated by a positive pressure ventilator. The abdominal contents then move the diaphragm upwards, causing a forced exsufflation. With bladder deflation the abdominal contents and diaphragm fall to the resting position as a result of gravity and inspiration occurs passively. Since the passive inspiration is dependent on gravity to return the diaphragm to its pre-bladder insufflation position, a trunk angle of 30° or more from the horizontal is necessary for adequate tidal volumes to occur. If the patient has any inspiratory capacity or is capable of effective GPB, he can add his autonomous tidal volume to the mechanically assisted inspiration.

The Switch to Tracheostomy IPPV

Trendelenburg was the first to describe the use of a tracheostomy tube with an inflated cuff for assisting ventilation during anesthesia of a human in 1869 (19). The use of transoral intubation for ventilatory support during anesthesia was described soon afterwards (20). In 1893 a hand-powered bellows was devised for delivering IPPV. Rubber tubing connected it to the patient either through a tight-fitting oral-nasal interface or a tracheostomy tube (21,22). Tracheostomy and the use of a mechanical bellows for ventilatory support were popularized for use with anesthesia during World War I (23). Despite its use for anesthesia and the fact that tracheostomies were not infrequently placed for the management of airway secretions in patients ventilated by iron lungs and other body ventilators in the 1940s, tracheostomy tubes were not used for chronic ventilatory support before the inadequate supply of body ventilators made this a necessity during the Danish poliomyelitis epidemic in 1952 (24). Although body ventilators had been adequate to ventilate patients, the patients were immobilized by them. Evacuation of respiratory tract secretions was very difficult for these patients without tracheostomy and with limited or no access to the body for manual-assisted coughing. Noninvasive intermittent positive airway pressure ventilatory support had not yet been reported, and mechanical forced exsufflation devices for effective evacuation of airway secretions were not available until after 1953 (25,28). Tracheostomy IPPV, therefore, gradually became the most popular for long-term ventilatory support after 1952.

Numerous reports have since appeared on complications related to tracheostomy and long-term tracheostomy IPPV (29). The complications have included nosocomial pneumonia (30-33), cardiac arrhythmias (34-36), and death from accidental disconnection despite alarms (37,38). Gram negative bacterial colonization (30) is common, as well as mucus plugging, chronic purulent bronchitis, granulation formation, and sepsis from stomal infection or paranasal sinusitis (39,40). Tracheostomy tube wall or cuff mucus plugs may be impossible to clear by suctioning and can fall into a bronchus and cause cardiopulmonary arrest. Other complications include tracheomalacia and tracheal perforation, hemorrhage, and tracheal stenosis, which occurs in 17-65 percent of patients (41), tracheoesophageal fistula (42), painful hemorrhagic tube changes, and psychosocial disturbances. The presence of a tracheostomy tube stimulates bronchial secretions, necessitates regular bronchial suctioning and routine toilet of the site as well as regular changing of the tube and ventilator tubing itself. Supplemental humidification must be provided and attended to daily. Speech is dependent on the cycling ventilator, and GPB is rarely effective. Swallowing problems and food aspiration may also occur (43). In addition to these difficulties, in many states the tracheostomy is considered an open wound, which may prevent community living without prohibitively expensive nursing care for tracheal suctioning, etc. Some schools and places of employment also prohibit patients with "open wounds."

Electrophrenic Respiration

The effect of electrical stimulation of the phrenic nerve on diaphragm motion was first recorded over 200 years ago by Caldani (44). Numerous reports of resuscitation by restoration of respiration using electrical stimulation of the phrenic nerve followed (45,46). Despite its success in resuscitation, stimulation of the phrenic nerves was discontinued as a method of artificial respiration when methods for negative pressure ventilatory support became available (45). Then, in 1948, Sarnoff and his associates demonstrated that adequate ventilation could be obtained by unilateral stimulation of the phrenic nerve (47). In 1968, Glenn and Judson (48) reported a case in which they used a permanently implantable system for electrical stimulation of the phrenic nerve. They successfully used EPR on an intermittent long-term basis for a patient with primary hypoventilation. Since 1972, about 700 phrenic nerve pacers have been implanted to provide ventilatory support in patients with central hypoventilation, chronic obstructive pulmonary disease, and high level quadriplegia, with variable success (49-54).

EPR consists of the transmission of a radio-wave signal by an antenna placed on the skin to an implanted receiver. The signal is converted to electrical impulses which are carried to electrodes in contact with the phrenic nerves. The impulses are delivered in a manner which simulates the natural recruitment of phrenic nerve fibers to stimulate the diaphragm. The indications for EPR are essentially limited to high level quadriplegics and patients with severe central hypoventilation with intact phrenic nerves and diaphragmatic function. Problems, however, include operative risks, infection, and trauma to the easily damaged phrenic nerves. The in-hospital training period is 6 to 16 weeks, frequently much longer, and the total expenses exceed $100,000. Unilateral pacing causes paradoxical diaphragmatic movement and possibly microatelectasis. Tidal volumes cannot be routinely modified, and voice quality is poorer than for patients using noninvasive methods of support, especially when those methods are supplemented by GPB. EPR patients are also subject to potential complications from their tracheostomy. A tracheostomy usually needs to be maintained because of the upper airway collapse that occurs during sleep on EPR and because of not uncommon sudden operational failure (55). This is particularly dangerous because of the lack of internal alarms and the inability to use GPB effectively. Infection can also occur with long-term use. Neuromuscular fatigue not infrequently leads to irreparable phrenic nerve and diaphragm damage (55,56).

Noninvasive Direct Airway-Supported Ventilation

Noninvasive intermittent positive airway pressure ventilatory support for the alert, cooperative patient was first reported in 1969, however, its use had begun over a decade earlier (57). Air is delivered to the patient through the mouth (11,58-60), nose (61-63), or mouth and nose (64-66) through appropriate patient ventilator interfaces.

In the mid- to late-1950s many patients dependent upon body ventilators learned to use mouth IPPV to supplement their body ventilator assisted volumes, especially for more effective coughing during respiratory tract infections. Mouth IPPV was also used for daytime support to free patients from their confining tank ventilators. Dr. Alba discovered that as patients would nap during the daytime, the mouth piece generally did not fall out of their mouths and ventilation was assisted despite their being asleep. By 1964 a number of patients had already switched from nocturnal body ventilator use to mouth IPPV (11,58,60). Mouth IPPV permitted these patients to conveniently continue total ventilatory support without being subjected to a tracheostomy. Portable positive pressure ventilators became available with the Bantam (available from Lifecare Co., Lafayette, CO) in 1957. This increased the likelihood of patient discharge into the community. With the advent of the Bennett lip seal (Puritan-Bennett, Boulder, CO) in 1969, mouth IPPV could be delivered during sleep with less insufflation leak around the mouth piece and little risk of the mouth piece falling out of the mouth). In 1978 portable volume ventilators became available with the option of producing regular deep inspirations (sighs) and with a battery of safety alarms and other features. Over 100 patients have recently been reported to rely on mouth IPPV, either alone or in combination with body ventilators for 24-hour ventilatory support for up to 40 years (11,58,60).

In 1982, as an alternative to mouth IPPV for French muscular dystrophy patients, DeLaubier and her group were probably the first to attempt nasal IPPV (67). Commercially available nasal continuous positive airway pressure (CPAP) masks were used to deliver IPPV. Nasal bridge pressure and insufflation leak into the eyes were common complaints of these patients.

Attempts at nocturnal nasal IPPV and at customizing nasal interfaces were first described in 1987 (68). Custom molded nasal interfaces can now be obtained both commercially (SEFAM Company, distributed by Lifecare, Inc., Lafayette, CO) and individually in New Jersey (64,65) and in France (69).

Oral-nasal interfaces were described for long-term supported ventilation in 1989 (66). The interfaces used strap retention systems like those used for mouth or nasal IPPV. However, since effective ventilatory support could be provided by either nasal or mouth IPPV, or when necessary, mouth IPPV with the nose plugged by a clip or by cotton pledgets and tape, strap retained oral-nasal interfaces have not been widely used. Strapless oral-nasal interfaces with bite-plate retention have been used in Europe since 1985 but were first described in the medical literature in 1989 (65). These interfaces not only provide an essentially hermetic seal for the delivery of IPPV, but simple tongue thrust is all that is necessary to expel them in the event of vomiting or other need. The bite-plate retention is important for patients living alone who are unable to don straps because of limited upper extremity range of motion or strength (70).

All three methods can be used for daytime as well as for nocturnal ventilatory support and are being given increasing attention in the medical literature. Although the intermittent abdominal pressure ventilator is the ventilator of choice for daytime support, it is not always effective, particularly in the presence of severe scoliosis. Daytime mouth IPPV is then generally indicated. Daytime nasal IPPV is indicated only for patients who can not retain a mouth piece in their mouths because of oral muscle weakness or inadequate jaw opening. It is also indicated when patients do not have sufficient neck rotation to grab a mouth piece held near the mouth (60).

Ventilation delivered by noninvasive methods of ventilatory support can be supplemented by the use of glossopharyngeal breathing (60). This technique was first recognized and described in the early 1950s (71,72). It can permit an otherwise totally ventilator-dependent patient up to hours of time free off his or her ventilator, but it is difficult if not impossible to use effectively in the presence of a tracheostomy.

MANAGEMENT OF AIRWAY SECRETIONS

Most paralytic/restrictive ventilator-dependent patients have difficulty in coughing and clearing airway secretions. Special attention is required for patients using noninvasive aids who have respiratory tract infections. Airway suctioning via the nose or mouth is not very effective and is poorly tolerated. As noted, tracheostomies have been placed for the sole purpose of aspiration of airway secretions. Tracheal suctioning, however, causes irritation, increases secretions, and may be accompanied by severe hypoxia

(73) and possibly cardiac arrhythmia. The suction catheter will usually not enter the left main-stem bronchus and will therefore not help to clear the left bronchial tree (74). Tracheal suctioning is at best effective at clearing only proximal pulmonary secretions and is ineffective in clearing life-threatening mucous plugs which adhere between the tracheostomy tube and tracheal wall and cuff. Suctioning can effectively be replaced in many circumstances by mouth IPPV with "air stacking," manual or mechanical assisted coughing, and postural drainage (75). Further, a mechanical forced exsufflation device can be used to clear pulmonary secretions.

The mechanical forced exsufflation device (Cof-flator) was described and extensively studied in 1953 and 1954 (25,28). This device delivers a deep, adjustable insufflation via an oral-nasal interface which is immediately followed by an independently adjustable exsufflation caused by a sudden drop in pressure from approximately 40 mm Hg to approximately -40 mm Hg in 0.2 seconds. This negative pressure is set to be sustained for 1.5 to 2 seconds. It generates 5 to 10 liters/sec of expiratory flow which is adequate for effective clearance of airway secretions. Clearance of secretions in this manner is less labor intensive and more effective than using manual-assisted coughing or tracheal suctioning through the mouth or nose. Many ventilator-dependent patients with inadequate cough continue to use this device to clear airway secretions during respiratory tract infections. Although safe and effective, manufacture of this device was discontinued soon after it was introduced because of the widespread use of tracheostomy tubes for tracheal suctioning and supported ventilation. It was nonetheless available for rental until the absence of replacement parts made this unfeasible in 1988. Its wider application today, however, would be strongly indicated for many patients with ineffective cough, whether dependent on ventilatory assistance or not. We are currently evaluating the prototype of a new mechanical forced exsufflation device.

FUTURE CONSIDERATIONS

Although negative pressure body ventilators have been successfully used by carbon dioxide retaining, chronic obstructive pulmonary disease patients (76-78), prolonged expiratory times and air trapping create difficulties when assisting the ventilation of these patients, and no negative pressure equivalent to CPAP is currently available. New negative pressure ventilator designs, such as the Negavent series (Lifecare, Inc., Lafayette, CO) and other as yet unnamed ventilators (Emerson Co., Cambridge, MA) are being designed to address the difficulties. These ventilators include the options of assist control negative extrathoracic pressure assisted ventilation, which should improve the ventilator's capture of the patient's breathing rhythm, and continuous negative extrathoracic pressure. This is the negative pressure equivalent of the mechanical effects of CPAP and is designed to have the same clinical applications. Interestingly, both CPAP and continuous negative extrathoracic pressure were first described in the 1870s (79,80).

The Negavent series ventilators are also being designed to have the capacity to follow the negative pressure cycle with an expiratory positive pressure cycle. When used in conjunction with a strapped-on Chest Shell or a Porta-lung, this should assist not only the inspiratory phase but decrease expiratory time, as well. With the accurate monitoring of pressure by having a pressure sensor which extends from the ventilator hose under the shell, wrap, or cylinder, this ventilator can compensate for wrap air leakage. The Emerson machine will also have a separate positive pressure sensor which can be placed in the ventilator circuit of a positive pressure ventilator while using simultaneously a negative pressure body ventilator and noninvasive positive airway assisted ventilation. Cessation of positive pressure from the positive pressure ventilator will trigger the Emerson ventilator, thus synchronizing the simultaneous use of both modalities. Simultaneous use of a rocking bed or iron lung with nose IPPV or mouth IPPV has been particularly useful in managing patients with paralytic/restrictive respiratory failure during respiratory tract infections (61), but synchronizing the actions has thus far been difficult.

Low- and high-pressure alarms, among other alarms, have been incorporated into positive pressure or volume ventilators over the last 20 years. Although useful for patients on IPPV via tracheostomy, the alarms complicate the use of daytime mouth IPPV and nasal IPPV and may hinder the patient's becoming accustomed to noninvasive airway intermittent positive pressure ventilatory support during sleep. They also add weight to the ventilator. The Zephyr (available from Lifecare, Inc., Lafayette, CO), which has been available since the 1950s, is a simple continuous blower which has been used by patients for sighing and for mouth IPPV during daytime hours. Absence of a cycling mechanism makes it impractical for sleep. There has been a recent effort to produce simpler ventilators for noninvasive aids. The BiPAP (Respironics, Monroeville, PA) is one such machine. It is essentially a pressure-limited blower up to a pressure of 15 cm H_2O with delivered volumes plateauing at greater pressures (81). The BiPAP weighs only 12 pounds and is useful for air delivery without high- and low-pressure alarms. The absence of alarms is generally not a problem for the patient population because the most appropriate alarm systems when necessary for patients on mouth or nose IPPV are not pressure alarms but alarms based on oxygen desaturation or elevations of end-tidal PCO_2 during sleep.

In summary, technological advances have increased the safety and portability of both positive and negative pressure ventilators over the last 30 years. The machines drive an ever increasing variety of available body ventilators and permit the use of noninvasive positive airway pressure ventilatory aids. We expect that new mechanical forced exsufflation devices will also be manufactured. Such advances give realistic hopes to patients with chronic alveolar hypoventilation for maintenance of adequate ventilation without the encumbrance of a tracheostomy, and thus for a significantly better quality of life. They also optimize the possibilities for patients to return to their homes.

The author would like to acknowledge the assistance of Dr. Augusta Alba for what was gleaned from her wealth of knowledge about the early forms of nontracheostomy positive pressure ventilation.

NOTES

1. Stover, S.L., P.R. Fine, and E.J. Kennedy, eds., *Spinal Cord Injury: The Facts and Figures* (Birmingham, AL: The University of Alabama, 1986), pp. 57–59.

2. Wilcos, N.E., and S. Stauffer, "Follow-up of 423 Consecutive Patients Admitted to the Spinal Cord Centre, Rancho Los Amigos Hospital, 1 January to 31 December 1967," *Paraplegia* 1972;10:115–122.

3. Gilroy, J., J.L. Cahalan, R. Berman, and M. Newman, "Cardiac Complications in Duchenne's Progressive Muscular Dystrophy," *Circulation* 1963;27:484–493.

4. Gordon, A.S., "History and Evolution of Modern Resuscitation Techniques," in A.S. Gordon, ed., *Cardiopulmonary Resuscitation Conference Proceedings* (Washington, DC: National Academy of Sciences, 1966):7–32.

5. Hill, N.S., "Clinical Applications of Body Ventilators," *Chest* 1986;90: 897–905.

6. Dalziel, J., "On Sleep and an Apparatus for Promoting Artificial Respiration," *Br Assoc Advancement Sci* 1838;2:127.

7. Woollam, C.H.M., "The Development of Apparatus for Intermittent Negative Pressure Respiration (1) 1832–1918," *Anaesthesia* 1976;31:537–547.

8. Emerson, J.H., and J.A. Loynes, *The Evolution of Iron Lungs: Respirators of the Body-Encasing Type* (Cambridge, MA: J. H. Emerson Company, 1978).

9. Eve, F.G., "Actuation of Inert Diaphragm by Gravity Method," *Lancet* 1932;2:995–997.

10. Bryce-Smith, R., and H.S. Davis, "Tidal Exchange in Respirators," *Curr Res Anaesth and Analges* 1954;33:73–85.

11. Bach, J.R., A.S. Alba, G. Bohatiuk, L. Saporito, and M. Lee, "Mouth Intermittent Positive Pressure Ventilation in the Management of Postpolio Respiratory Insufficiency," *Chest* 1987;91:859–864.

12. The Council on Physical Medicine, "Acceptability of the Fairchild-Huxley Cuirass Respirator," *JAMA* 1950;143:1157.

13. The Council on Physical Medicine, "The Monaghan Portable Respirator Acceptance Report," *JAMA* 1949;139:1273.

14. Bach, J.R., and A.S. Alba, "Total Ventilatory Support by the Intermittent Abdominal Pressure Ventilator," *Chest* (submitted for publication).

15. Spalding, J.M.K., and L. Opiel, "Artificial Respiration With the Tunnicliffe Breathing Jacket," *Lancet* 1958;274:613–615.

16. Bach, J.R., and F. Beltrame, "Alternative Methods of Ventilatory Support," in M.M. Rothkopf and J. Askanazi, eds., *Home Intensive Care* (Baltimore: Williams & Wilkins, in press).

17. McSweeney, C.J., "The Bragg-Paul Pulsator in Treatment of Respiratory Paralysis," *Br Med J* 1938;1:1206–1207.

18. Adamson, J.P., L. Lewis, and J.D. Stein, "Application of Abdominal Pressure for Artificial Respiration," *JAMA* 1959;169: 153–157.

19. Trendelenburg, F., "Beitrage zur den Operationen an den Luftwagen 2, Tamponnade der Trachea," *Arch Klin Chir* 1871:12:121–233.

20. MacEwen, W., "Clinical Observations on the Introduction of Tracheal Tubes by the Mouth Instead of Performing Tracheotomy or Laryngotomy," *Br Med J* 1880;2:122–124.

21. Hochberg, L.A., *Thoracic Surgery before the 20th Century* (New York: Vantage Press, 1960), pp. 684–697.

22. Fell, G.E., "Forced Respiration," *JAMA* 1891;16:325–330.

23. Magill, I.W., "Development of Endotracheal Anesthesia," *Proc R Soc Med* 1928;22:83–88.

24. Lassen, H.C.A., "The Epidemic of Poliomyelitis in Copenhagen, 1952," *Proc R Soc Med* 1954;47:67–71.

25. "The OEM Cof-flator Portable Cough Machine," Shampaine Industries, Inc, St. Louis, MO.

26. Barach, A.L., G.J. Beck, H.A. Bickerman, and H.E. Seanor, "Physical Methods Simulating Cough Mechanisms," *JAMA* 1952;150: 1380–1385.

27. Barach, A.L., G.J. Beck, and R.H. Smith, "Mechanical Production of Expiratory Flow Rates Surpassing the Capacity of Human Coughing," *Amer J Med Sci* 1953;226:241–248.

28. Bickerman, H.A., and S. Itkin, "Exsufflation With Negative Pressure," *Arch Int Med* 1954;93: 698–704.

29. Bellamy, R., F.W. Pitts, and S. Stauffer, "Respiratory Complications in Traumatic Quadriplegia," *J Neurosurg* 1973;39:596–600.

30. Niederman, M.S., R.D. Ferranti, A. Ziegler, W. Merrill, and H.Y. Reynolds, "Respiratory Infection Complicating Long-term Tracheostomy: The Implication of Persistent Gram-negative Tracheobronchial Colonization," *Chest* 1984;85:39–44.

31. Johanson, W.G., A.K. Pierce, J.P. Sanford, and G.D. Thomas, "Nosocomial Respiratory Infections With Gram-negative Bacilli: The Significance of Colonization of the Respiratory Tract," *Ann Int Med* 1972;77:701–706.

32. Johanson, W.G., J.J. Seidenfeld, P. Gomez, R. De Los Santos, and J.J. Coalson, "Bacteriologic Diagnosis of Nosocomial Pneumonia Following Prolonged Mechanical Ventilation," *Am Rev Respir Dis* 1988;137:259–264.

33. Craven, D.E., L.M. Kunches, V. Kilinsky, D.A. Lichtenberg, B.J. Make, and W.R. McCabe, "Risk Factors for Pneumonia and Fatality in Patients Receiving Continuous Mechanical Ventilation," *Am Rev Respir Dis* 1986;133:792–796.

34. Berk, J.L., and M.N. Levy, "Profound Reflex Bradycardia Produced by Transient Hypoxia or Hypercapnia in Man," *Eur Surg Res* 1977;9:75–84.

35. Mathias, C.J., "Bradycardia and Cardiac Arrest During Tracheal Suction—Mechanisms in Tetraplegic Patients," *Europ J Intens Care Med* 1976;2:147–156.

36. Welply, N.C., C.J. Mathias, and H.L. Frankel, "Circulatory Reflexes in Tetraplegics During Artificial Ventilation and General Anesthesia," *Paraplegia* 1975;13: 172–182.

37. Splaingard, M.L., R.C. Frates, G.M. Harrison, R.E. Carter, and L.S. Jefferson, "Home Positive-pressure Ventilation: Twenty Years' Experience," *Chest* 1984;4:376–382.

38. Bach, J.R., and A.S. Alba, "Management of Chronic Alveolar Hypoventilation by Nasal Ventilation," *Chest* 1990;97:52–57.

39. Moar, J.J., G.E. Lello, and S.D. Miller, "Stomal Sepsis and Fatal Haemorrhage Following Tracheostomy," *Int J Oral Maxillofac Surg* 1986;15:339–341.

40. Deutschman, C.S., P. Wilton, J. Sinow, D. Dibbell, F.N. Konstantinides, and F.B. Cerra, "Paranasal Sinusitis Associated With Nasotracheal Intubation: A Frequently Unrecognized and Treatable Source Of Sepsis," *Crit Care Med* 1986;14: 111–114.

41. Pingleton, S.K., "Complications of Acute Respiratory Failure," *Am Rev Respir Dis* 1988;37:1463–1493.

42. Hedden, M., C. Ersoz, and P. Safar, "Tracheoesophageal Fistulas Following Prolonged Artificial Ventilation Via Cuffed Tracheostomy Tubes," *Anesthesiology* 1969;31:281–289.

43. Bonanno, P., "Swallowing Dysfunction After Tracheostomy," *Ann Surg* 1971;174:29–33.

44. Caldani, L.M.A., *Institutiones Physiologicae* (Venezia: Pezzana, 1786), cited by D.C. Schecter, "Application of Electrotherapy to Non-cardiac Disorders," *Bull NY Acad Med* 1970;46:932–951.

45. Glenn, W.O.O.L., and M.L. Phelps, "Diaphragmatic Pacing by Electrical Stimulation of the Phrenic Nerve," *Neurosurg* 1985;17:974–984.

46. Duchenne, G., *De l'electrisation localisée et de son application à la pathologic et à la thérapeutique* (Paris: Baillière, 1872): 914. Cited in R.G. Vanderlinden, S.W. Epstein, R.H. Hyland, H.S. Smythe, and L.D. Vanderlinden, "Management of Chronic Ventilatory Insufficiency With Electrical Diaphragm Pacing," *Can J Neuro Sci* 1988;15:63–67.

47. Sarnoff, S.J., E. Hardenbergh, and J.L. Whittenberger, "Electrophrenic Respiration," *Am J Physiol* 1948;155: 1–9.

48. Judson, J.P., and W.O.O.L. Glenn, "Radiofrequency Electrophrenic Respiration: Long-term Application to a Patient With Primary Hypoventilation," *JAMA* 1968;203:1033–1037.

49. Glenn, W.O.O.L., W.G. Holcomb, A.J. McLaughlin, J.M. O'Hare, J.F. Hogan, and R. Yasuda, "Total Ventilatory Support in Quariplegic Patient With Radiofrequency Electrophrenic Respiration," *N Engl J Med* 1972;286:513–516.

50. Glenn, W.O.O.L., J.F. Hogan, J.S.O. Loke, T.E. Ciesielski, M.L. Phelps, and R. Rowedder, "Ventilatory Support by Pacing of Conditioned Diaphragm in Quadriplegia," *N Engl J Med* 1984;310:1150–1155.

51. Glenn, W.O.O.L., J.F. Hogan, and M.L. Phelps, "Ventilatory Support of Quadriplegic Patient With Respiratory Paralysis by Diaphragm Pacing," *Surg Clinic North Am* 1980;60: 1055–1078.

52. Glenn, W.O.O.L., W.G. Holcomb, R.K. Shaw, J.F. Hogan, and K.R. Holschuh, "Long-term Ventilatory Support by Diaphragm Pacing in Quadriplegia," *Ann Surg* 1976:183:566–576.

53. Stauffer, E.S., and G.D. Bell, "Traumatic Respiratory Quadriplegia and Pentaplegia," *Orthop Clin North Am* 1978;9:1081–1089.

54. Glenn, W.O.O.L., J.B.L. Gee, and E.N. Schacter, "Diaphragm Pacing: Application to a Patient With Chronic Obstructive Pulmonary Disease," *J Thorac Cardiovasc Surg* 1978;75:273–281.

55. Oakes, D.D., C.B. Wilmot, D. Halverson, and R.D. Hamilton, "Neurogenic Respiratory Failure: A 5-year Experience Using Implantable Phrenic Nerve Stimulators," *Ann Thorac Surg* 1980;30:118–122.

56. McMichan, J.C., D.G. Piepgras, D.R. Gracey, H.M. Marsh, and R. Sittipong, "Electrophrenic Respiration," *Mayo Clin Proc* 1979;54: 662–668.

57. Alba, A., M. Solomon, and F.S. Trainor, "Management of Respiratory Insufficiency in Spinal Cord Lesions," in *Proceedings of the 17th Veteran's Administration Spinal Cord Injury Conference, 1969,* U.S. Government Printing Office 0-436-398, 1971:200–213.

58. Bach, J., J. O'Brien, R. Krotenberg, and A. Alba, "Management of End Stage Respiratory Failure in Patients With Duchenne Muscular Dystrophy," *Muscle & Nerve* 1987;10: 177–182.

59. Curran, F.J., and A.P. Colbert, "Ventilator Management in Duchenne Muscular Dystrophy and Postpoliomyelitis Syndrome: Twelve Years' Experience," *Arch Phys Med Rehabil* 1989: 70;180–185.

60. Bach, J.R., A.S. Alba, E. Bodofsky, F.J. Curran, and M. Schultheiss, "Glossopharyngeal Breathing and Non-invasive Aids in the Management of Post-polio Respiratory Insufficiency," *Birth Defects* 1987;23:99–113.

61. Bach, J.R., and A.S. Alba, "Management of Chronic Alveolar Hypoventilation by Nasal Ventilation," *Chest* 1990;97:52–57.

62. Ellis, E.R., P.T.P. Bye, J.W. Bruderer, and C.E. Sullivan, "Treatment of Respiratory Failure During Sleep in Patients With Neuromuscular Disease: Positive-pressure Ventilation Through a Nose Mask," *Amer Rev Respir Dis* 1987;135:148–152.

63. Kerby, G.R., L.S. Mayer, and S.K. Pingleton, "Nocturnal Positive Pressure Ventilation Via Nasal Mask," *Am Rev Respir Dis* 1987;135:738–740.

64. Bach, J.R., A.S. Alba, and D. Shin, "Noninvasive Airway Pressure Assisted Ventilation in the Management of Respiratory Insufficiency Due to Poliomyelitis," *Amer J Phys Med Rehabil* 1989;68:264–271.

65. McDermott, I., J.R. Bach, C. Parker, and S. Sortor, "Custom-fabricated Interfaces for Intermittent Positive Pressure Ventilation," *Int J Prosthodont* 1989;2:224–233.

66. Ratzka, A., "Uberdruckbeatmung durch Mundstuck," in U. Frehse, ed., *Spatfolgen nach Poliomyelitis: Chronische Unterbeatmung und Moglichkeiten selbstbestimmter Lebensfuhrung Schwerbehinderter* (Munchen: Pfennigparade eV, 1989);5:149.

67. Delaubier, A., "Traitement de l'insuffisance respiratoire chronique dans les dystrophies musculaires," in *Memoires de certificat d'etudes superieures de reeducation et readaptation fonctionnelles* (Paris: Universite R Descarte, 1984):1–124.

68. Bach, J.F., A. Alba, R. Mosher, and A. Delaubier, "Intermittent Positive Pressure Ventilation Via Nasal Access in the Management of Respiratory Insufficiency," *Chest* 1987;92:168–170.

69. Leger, P., J. Jennequin, M. Gerard, and D. Robert, "Home Positive Pressure Ventilation Via Nasal Mask for Patients With Neuromuscular Weakness or Restrictive Lung or Chest-wall Disease," *Resp Care* 1989;34:73–79.

70. Bach, J.R., and I. McDermott, "Strapless Oral-nasal Interfaces for Positive Pressure Ventilation," *Arch Phys Med Rehabil* (in press).

71. Dail, C., M. Rodgers, V. Guess, and H.V. Adkins, *Glossopharyngeal Breathing Manual* (Downey, CA: Professional Staff Assoc. of Rancho Los Amigos Hospital, Inc, 1979).

72. Dail, C.W., and J.E. Affeldt, "Glossopharyngeal Breathing" (video) (Los Angeles, Department of Visual Education, College of Medical Evangelists, 1954).

73. Bach, J.R., S. Sortor, and M. Sipski, "Sleep Blood Gas Monitoring of High Cervical Quadriplegic Patients With Respiratory Insufficiency by Non-invasive Techniques" (abs), *Abstracts Digest,* 14th Annual Scientific Meeting of the American Spinal Cord Injury Association, p. 102. Available from L. H. Johnson, 2020 Peachtree Road, NW, Atlanta, GA, 1988.

74. Fishhurn, M.J., R.J. Marino, and J.F. Ditunno, "Atelectasis and Pneumonia in Acute Spinal Cord Injury," *Arch Phys Med Rehabil* 1990;71:197–200.

75. Sortor, S., and M. McKenzie, "Toward Independence: Assisted Cough" (video) (BioScience Communications of Dallas, Inc, 1986).

76. Braun, N.M.T., and W.D. Marino, "Effect of Daily Intermittent Rest of Respiratory Muscles in Patients With Severe Chronic Airflow Limitation," *Chest* 1984;85:59s.

77. Cropp, A., and A.F. DiMarco, "Effects of Intermittent Negative Pressure Ventilation on Respiratory Muscle Function in Patients With Severe Chronic Obstructive Disease," *Am Rev Respir Dis* 1987;135: 1056–1061.

78. Ambrosino, N., T. Montagni, A. Negri, S. Brega, C. Fracchia, and C. Rampulla, "Negative Pressure Ventilation Induces Long Term Improve-

ment of Exercise Tolerance of COPD Patients" [Abstract], *Eur Resp J* 1989;2:363s.

79. Von Hauke, I., *Der Pneumatische Panzer. Beitrag zur "mechanischen Behandlung der Brustkrankheiten"* (Wiener: Medizinische Presse 1874):15:785,836.

80. Waldenburg, L., *Die pneumatische Behandlung der Respirations und Circulationskrankheiten im Anschluss an die Pneumatometrie und Spirometrie* (Berlin: Hirschwald, 1880):420.

81. Strumpf, D.A.,C.C. Carlisle, R.P. Millman, and N.S. Hill, "Bi-level Positive Airway Pressure (BiPAP): A Low-cost, Simple Method of Providing Nocturnal Assisted Ventilation," *Am Rev Respir Dis* [abstract] 1989;139:A155.

26

AN ASTRONAUT ON EARTH

Paul Kahn

In November 1987 I underwent a tracheotomy and became permanently wedded to a ventilator. In this narrative I shall trace the circumstances that led to that intervention and explain my anticipatory anxieties about how it might reduce the quality of my life. I shall also describe my physical and psychological recovery. And, in particular, I shall discuss the internal and external resources that helped me cope with the traumatic change and enabled me to resume a satisfying lifestyle.

Though painful and challenging, this ordeal also taught me valuable insights about self-determination and the ability of the psyche to incorporate and adapt to new realities. I shall try to pass on these insights in the hope that others faced with the need for a tracheotomy will benefit from them and feel more optimistic about their prospects.

I had a tracheotomy because I was no longer able to breathe adequately on my own. The inability was the endpoint of a long decline caused by my centronuclear myopathy, a congenital, progressive neuromuscular disability. For many years I had been getting ventilation at night by means of a positive pressure respirator that fed air to me through a lip-sealed mouthpiece. During the day I was able to breathe on my own well enough to do things that mattered to me: work, art, and socializing.

Gradually, as my breathing muscles weakened, I began to need more assistance during the day. I started using oxygen from a liquid oxygen tank. Then I began having to use a respirator for an hour in the late afternoon. The hour became insufficient and the year before my tracheotomy, I needed extended and repeated intervals on the respirator throughout the day. Even so, I was always tired. Any exercise, mental or physical, exhausted me and required great willpower. I lost weight because I did not have the energy to eat. My life was measured and restricted by the few hours of relative comfort I experienced before cyanosis forced me to return to the respirator.

Fearful and desperate, I had myself admitted into the respiratory care center of a large Boston hospital, where the pressure of carbon dioxide in my blood was found to range between 90 and 100. I was told that this was a life-threatening situation and that the only reason I was not dead was that over the years my body had gradually adjusted to unnaturally high CO_2 levels. I felt that, if not technically dead, I was certainly not alive in the way I wanted to be. My existence seemed a hopeless, dreary nursing of my invalidism. I could not continue that way.

I had suffered with my deteriorating health for two reasons. One, I nurtured the fantasy that I would get better on my own. I had experienced bouts of respiratory failure before yet had always recovered to a functional status. I thought that if I coddled myself and was patient enough, I would do so again. My rational mind understood that my primary disability was progressive, the slide toward loss inexorable, but emotionally I wanted to believe that my willpower could enable me to live and thrive. I proudly remembered one of my doctors writing in a report that he had never seen anyone who had accomplished so much in the face of such severe limitations. To give in to the tracheotomy meant compromising this belief in my special powers. It also meant acknowledging and having to reconcile myself to my physical deterioration, my mortality.

The second reason I did not seek a tracheotomy earlier was that I was afraid both of the operation and the outcome. As long as I can recall, I have been deeply distrustful of other people, while having to depend on them for my basic needs. The struggle to achieve some measure of self-reliance has been central to my life. To lie unconscious on the operating table and let masked strangers hold my life in their latex-gloved hands seemed the antithesis of this desired self-reliance.

I was also afraid of how the operation might change the quality of my life. Being completely dependent on a ventilator, would I always feel anxious about it breaking down? Would I ever again be able to enjoy the peace of solitude or would I always need to have someone hovering around me to provide emergency aid in case of such break-downs? Would other people be frightened or repulsed by my strange accouterments? In particular, how would my new girlfriend, Ruth, feel? Would she continue to find me attractive? And, how would I feel about myself? Being so intimately, so inextricably joined to a machine, would I feel less human—like a robot instead of a flesh-and-blood man? The image came to me of a space-walking astronaut, tethered by a fragile umbilical line to his capsule. Never could he forget how deadly was the void in which he floated, how without his clumsy high-tech gadgetry he would die. I imagined seeing the strain of constant fear on his helmeted face. I wondered, would I be an astronaut on earth?

To help prepare for the tracheotomy, the respiratory care center showed me, my parents, and Ruth videotapes about patients who had undergone the procedure. They and the people intimately involved in their lives spoke about how they had adjusted and were coping. I felt reassured by their positive attitudes and by the fact that the tracheostomy tube and ventilator circuitry seemed aesthetically much less intrusive than I had imagined. The center staff, particularly Mary, the wise, warm, and earthy woman who served as associate director, did its best to answer our questions, although the answers were always too hedged with qualifications to be comforting. You will probably be able to resume your normal life, they said. You will probably be able to talk. The only thing they seemed completely sure about was that I would never be free of the ventilator again. Concerning the terrors of surgery and the anguish of confronting so many uncertainties, we were helped by Jennifer, a young chaplain who gave us her compassionate attention and made us feel safe enough to express our anxieties about what we might have to live through.

The surgery consisted of making an opening at the base of my throat into my trachea and inserting a curved, plastic tracheostomy tube, to which a ventilator was then attached. It went well, and the next morning Ruth and my parents were amazed to find me sitting up in my wheelchair, looking pinker and more energized than they had seen me in over a year.

However, there were unanticipated delays in my progress toward full recovery. Two disheartening problems were my inability to talk or eat for several weeks after the surgery. I could not talk because the staff decided that to ventilate me most efficiently the cuff on the tracheostomy tube had to be kept inflated. An inflated cuff prevents the escape of air around the tube but, in doing so, it also prevents air from passing through the vocal cords, making speech impossible.

During this period I communicated first by spelling words on alphabet cards and then by learning to use an electro-larynx. Holding this device against my throat, I silently articulated and was able to produce a gravelly, indistinct, uninflected approximation of speech. Despite this aid, I felt endangered by not being able to effectively communicate my needs. The prospect of facing life without a voice was appalling. I had always been verbally oriented and took pride in being articulate. Talking was how I expressed my intellect and emotions. When people saw me after the surgery, would they see my disability and think me different? If they could hear me, they might understand and respect me. Also, as a psychotherapist, I depended on my voice. Not being able to speak would mean the end of my career.

Eventually the staff decided that I had stabilized enough for them to start deflating the cuff at intervals and let me practice speaking. This was challenging. It required me to reverse the normal pattern of speaking while exhaling. On a ventilator, you speak while air is being pumped in, using the flow that escapes around the tracheostomy tube and passes up through the vocal cords. The timing of inspiration and expiration is fixed, and the user cannot adjust it to create a natural flow of speech. My cycle was two seconds of inspiration and two seconds of expiration, which meant that every amount of available speaking time was abruptly intercut with an equal period of enforced silence, whether I was in the middle of a phrase or not. In my first uncoordinated attempts, I was able to get out just a few choppy words at a time; only with practice did I adjust and gain fluency.

However, it was a joy to speak at all, to sound like myself again. One of the first times I spoke was to answer a telephone call from Ruth. Expecting the mechanical sound of the electro-larynx, she was nonplussed when she heard my voice. "Is that really you?" she asked. "No," some impish impulse made me answer, "this is a recording." We both laughed, pleased and excited that an important medium of our intimacy had been reclaimed.

My delay in eating resulted from concerns that I would aspirate food and thereby develop respiratory infections. The surgical trauma to the throat and the introduction of the tracheostomy tube can often disrupt the swallowing mechanism, but this difficulty usually resolves itself after a few days. Mine did not. Every time the therapist tested me by giving me colored ice to swallow, some of it could be seen leaking out around my stoma, indicating that I had failed to direct it correctly into my esophagus. I had to be fed through a nasal-gastric tube. Naturally, I could not, and probably would not have wanted to, taste the thick, white nutritional liquid they pumped down it. This was a completely unpleasurable way to eat, and my repeated failures made me begin to despair of ever again enjoying the social and sensual pleasures of sharing a good meal with friends.

I remember particularly well being given a pass from the hospital on Thanksgiving, going to my parents' home, and having to sit and watch them and Ruth partake of turkey, stuffing, and all the usual (but to me forbidden) holiday delights. It was torture. And, if I cheated just a bit by dipping my finger into the gravy and tasting it, could I be blamed?

After three weeks with no improvement, the head physician of the center began to suspect that the presence of the nasal-gastric tube in my esophagus might be aggravating my swallowing difficulty. He decided to remove it and test how well I did without it. To my enormous relief, I passed. I was allowed to eat on my own again, though at first only the most nondescript, pureed food. Brown "mud" signified that it was some sort of meat, and green "mud" was some sort of vegetable. However, I quickly graduated to real food, which I devoured with a gusto based both on long deprivation and on the fact that I had the energy to eat again.

To celebrate our sixth month anniversary of going together, Ruth brought in a special meal she had purchased at a gourmet shop. We had lasagna, wine, and chocolate truffles for dessert. There was much to celebrate—the return of my health, the survival of our relationship—and yet much to feel anxious about. What, we wondered, would life be like at home with the ventilator, outside the security of the hospital?

Much of my stay at the hospital was devoted to getting ready for that transition. I realized that to regain my independence and feel comfortable in my apartment again, I would have to understand my new care needs and be able to teach them to my attendants. Also, Ruth and I knew that, if we were to have any privacy, she would have to learn everything, too. The operation of the ventilator had to be mastered, the meaning of its various settings and alarms, the method of disinfecting and changing its circuitry. Then there was the cleaning and protection of the stoma, the techniques of suctioning out bronchial secretions, and the maintenance of supplies such as catheters, drain sponges, and hydrogen peroxide.

We learned together, but the primary responsibility for mastering and being able to direct my care fell on me. I wanted it to, because I felt the need to be in charge of my life again. Luckily, when properly motivated, I can apply myself, and the learning posed no great difficulties. In fact, I found some enjoyment in acquiring the new skills, and the process gave a focus to my days that often seemed long and trying—I was working on going home.

Hospitalization was very stressful for me. In addition to the uncertainties about my recovery, I faced the anxiety of being dependent on a parade of strangers, who showed varying degrees of competence, kindness, and reliability. To minimize this dependence I tried as much as possible to bring my own familiar, reliable attendants into the hospital to assist me. But they could not be there at night or in the early morning, so those became my most insecure, homesick times.

Also, one-half of a small, bare hospital room was an impoverished environment to live in. I brought in books, games, art materials, writing materials, anything I thought would keep my mind active, but missed the comfort of my home and the stimulation of being out in the world. I remember two books that especially helped me bridge my isolation. One was *Psychotherapy: The Art of Wooing Nature,* a treatise by Sheldon Roth. It helped me feel that I had not entirely lost touch with my work, that, even though I was not practicing, I could still think about and improve my skills. The second was *Jitterbug Perfume,* a novel by Tom Robbins which dealt playfully and exuberantly with the search for immortality. It spoke to me because I had just thwarted death. Ruth and I were both comforted by its sweet insistence on the power of love and hope. We were so moved that we gave the name "Alobar," the hero of the novel, to a tiny but very hardy fly with whom I shared my room, and we invoked him as a guardian spirit. It seems silly in retrospect, but sometimes one has to create one's own myths in order to survive.

Probably the greatest stress of being in the hospital was the disruption of my relationship with Ruth. We had been going together for less than five months and were still in the first flush of wonder and pleasure at our intimacy. To be thrust into an environment that afforded us no privacy, no chance to escape from the compelling but abnormal drama of my recovery, seemed a great loss. We railed and grieved, but with Jennifer's help came to understand that the hospitalization was not an interruption in our relationship but a continuation of it. Once we had accepted that, we could open our eyes and appreciate the richness of our situation—my progress toward health, the sweetness of our kisses when that was all we could give each other, the support of our families and friends. We came to realize that wherever we were together could be our home.

That realization was the first spiritual lesson of the tracheotomy, the first answer to the questions I had asked myself about what the quality of my life would be. The quality would depend on me, on my attitude, not on my physical baggage or surroundings.

I entered the hospital on November 3, and 43 days later, on December 15, I was discharged. The chief resident's parting words to me were, "Congratulations on your new marriage to the ventilator. I'm sure that with your creativity you'll make the relationship work." I hoped so, but he had more faith in me than I had.

My parents shared my doubts. Many years before they had curbed their protective instincts and had not impeded me, their disabled son, from leaving the security of their care and starting an independent life in my own apartment. Now those instincts reasserted themselves, and my parents expressed fears about my living on my own again. They even suggested that they buy a two-family house and share it with me, so that they could be available, if I needed help. I was touched by their concern and their characteristic readiness to support me, but that degree of dependence seemed a giant step backwards that I had to refuse to take.

As I waited in the hospital lobby while my attendant, Jeff, loaded my van with my equipment and belongings, I noticed that the nearby admitting cubicles were doing a steady business. I felt sorry for the poor souls about to go through life-and-death dramas of their own and glad that I had emerged from mine. I went out into the crisp late autumn morning rejoicing about being a survivor. But on the way home anxiety overtook me. I became afraid that the ventilator hose might come loose from the tracheostomy tube, interrupting the flow of air on which I depended. Could I reattach the tube by myself? Could Jeff stop the van on the turnpike to help me? And how long could I breathe on my own, if I had to? I did not know the answers to these questions, so I held myself stiffly and prayed that the bouncing of the van would not shake anything loose. We got home without mishap and were met by therapists from the home care company, who had come to bring additional supplies, help me organize storage and equipment space, and clarify their services. I was glad of their competent presence and, when they left, again felt a dread. What now? I thought. Now I had to be the resident expert.

Gradually, my fears about equipment failure dissipated. With the ungrateful sarcasm we sometimes direct towards the people and things on which we are dependent, I called my ventilator a pretentious and overpriced air compressor, but I developed a grudging respect for and confidence in its intelligence, efficiency, and reliability. In addition to the one on the back of my wheelchair, I had a duplicate model beside my bed for nighttime use. I knew I could switch myself over to this second one, if something went wrong with the first. I also had my suction machine set up with a mirror, so that I could easily suction myself. I therefore felt quite safe being alone at home.

Away from home I always had to keep a manual ventilating device called an ambu bag with me for emergency use. Since I could not manipulate the bag myself, I needed to have someone close by who understood when and how to use it. I also always had to travel with other supplies, such as a portable suction machine and suction catheters. At first I worried that I would forget to take these necessities with me or forget to reorder supplies and run out. But stocking my travel bag and keeping up supplies eventually became an automatic rhythm like brushing one's teeth or paying rent. I also became adept at troubleshooting minor problems when they did occur, such as a cracked air filter or a loose connection in the circuitry.

So I learned to trust my equipment, but more importantly, I learned to trust myself. And that was the second lesson of the tracheotomy—the knowledge that I could be more mature than I thought. I could be responsible for my complex needs, and I could tolerate the degree of risk that was unavoidable if I wanted to live a full life. I began to see that my situation was not qualitatively different from anyone else's. If we want to drive anywhere, we must all trust that our brakes will hold and the bridges we ride over will not crumble beneath us, even though we know that brakes and bridges both occasionally give way. I take chances now that perhaps I should not, such as letting my attendant leave me for a few hours even when I am away from home. It is not that I am courageous. I am pragmatic, accepting the price of the ticket for my life.

When I first started going back into the world, I felt very conspicuous with the tracheostomy tube and ventilator. The experience was like becoming disabled all over again. A lifetime of using a wheelchair had accustomed me to stares and the quick, uncomfortable turning away of eyes. But in the last 15 years, improved access has made disabled people less of a rarity in public and decreased unwanted attention. Disabled people with ventilators are still a minority within a minority. I could not remember having seen any outside of institutions. I expected the world to greet me with a renewed onslaught of pity and fear, the old there-but-for-the-grace-of-God syndrome reborn in all its alienating force. Part of me wanted to avoid this confrontation and keep to the security of home. But I had struggled through the ordeal of the tracheotomy in order to have a fuller life, not a more curtailed one, so I ventured out.

Whether my predictions were accurate or not, I cannot say. How can we know other people's reality? To the significant people in my life, the tracheotomy seemed to matter little. My patients were simply glad that I was again able to attend to their problems. With the self-centeredness to which therapy gives complete permission, they were primarily concerned with how my condition might impact them. Once reassured that I was healthy and not going to die or leave them again, my patients were able to ignore my tracheotomy.

My colleagues were for the most part politely disinterested, a nonreaction that troubled me. I had, after all, gone through hell and back and, though I wanted to be regarded as essentially the same person I had always been, I also wanted some recognition of my ordeal and triumph—not so much a pat on the back as a little empathy.

I was grateful to those who were interested in hearing about my experience, who had the courage not to shrink from my tale of suffering. A few months after my tracheotomy I happened to meet an old friend, whom I had not seen for several years. She greeted me warmly and with great naturalness pointed to my ventilator. "That's new, isn't it?" she asked. She listened with interest as I told her what had happened, and when I was finished, she smiled and said, "It must have worked, because you look great. I'm glad for you." I thanked her for the compliment but was even more pleased by how comfortable she had made me feel. Hers was exactly the right reaction.

It was the kind of reaction I generally got from friends and family who loved me. They welcomed me back with relief and happiness. I embraced them and embraced the opportunities my new vitality afforded me. Everything I was able to do again felt so precious that my twinges of self-consciousness, my regret about having to carry around so much baggage, seemed less significant.

The formation of people's attitudes toward me and my self-concept has always seemed a reciprocal process. When I have projected self-respect, I have been granted respect. The tracheotomy upset my sense of identity. My bodily integrity felt violated, my fetal helplessness seemed confirmed. I needed to heal myself and feel whole again. I learned that the ways of self-healing I had used before still worked for me. One of the most important of these was artistic expression. By creating, giving visual or written form to my feelings, I have always felt able, through some sympathetic magic, to recreate myself.

I began putting this process to work while I was still in the hospital. The idea occurred to me of creating a mural to express the drama we were going through. My inspiration was Matisse, who in his old age was confined to bed and too arthritic to handle a paintbrush. So, he created collages by cutting shapes out of colored paper and directing his assistants where to place them on the wall in front of him. I modified his example by deciding that, instead of keeping autocratic control, I would let my assistants—Ruth and my attendants—be artistic partners and contribute to the design. It seemed only fair, since they were partners in my ordeal as well.

We began by laying in a supply of construction paper, scissors, tape, and glue and then covering most of one wall of my room with a large sheet of heavy white paper. I made a sketch of the area and divided it into three sections. The left I labeled "sickness," the center "recovery," and the right, "health." Together they would tell my story. To guide my collaborators and give some coherence to the design, I wrote down descriptive terms for each section. "Sickness" should be dark, cramped, sad, and weak. "Recovery" would be agitated, hopeful, and uncertain. And "health" must be bright, expansive, happy, strong, and free. We went to work and the blank wall slowly began to fill up with the shapes and colors of our imaginations. "Sickness" was covered with chains, bars, and ragged dark shapes. "Recovery" was dominated by a figure breaking out of the confines of a harsh, red box. "Health" climaxed the composition with multi-hued symbols of life and happiness—a winged man, a butterfly, lovers cradled by a crescent moon.

The progress of the mural paralleled my progress and was a powerful way of externalizing my tensions and, by doing so, dissipating some of their force. But, because of its collaborative, too loosely coordinated nature, the effort ultimately lacked the alchemical power of art to turn suffering into beauty. There are valuable parts of it that I will one day rework in more finished form. For now, though, the mural sits rolled up in my closet, waiting for the day when I have the courage to unwind the vivid memories it contains.

When I returned home, I continued to explore my experience in more finished work. The first painting I completed I called "Steppenwolf," after the novel by Hermann Hesse. The theme of the novel, the divided soul, seemed to mirror my own inner tensions and confusions. I was torn between rejoicing and regret: the rational adult in me knew to count his blessings of health, but the undisciplined child railed against the cost to his freedom and resented the burden of the limitations and responsibilities. I wavered between hope and dread: I might have life now, but death had come so close I could never feel completely safe again. And, I still did not know which to celebrate—the fury of my will to survive or the abeyance of my will and acceptance of the suffering that made survival possible. In the painting, these dualities were represented by the man and the wolf. By integrating these figures within a balanced, circular composition, I found a symbolic, ritualistic way of integrating and transcending my psychological conflicts.

As time passed and I grew more confident in my health, I felt able and compelled to revisit my pre-tracheotomy sickness. I vividly remembered my fatigue, my dread of dying, my dullness and emptiness, and I thought if I could make art out of that pain, I could triumph over it. The waste of those days could be transmuted into something I would be proud of, something that would touch and be valued by other people, too. The work that most directly realized that hope was a poem I called "Hollow Man."

Little pieces of disorder rebuke me.
In dry stacks unpaid bills
disdain my feckless, spendthrift ways.
Rotting leftovers reek of my slothfulness.
A cracked egg sheds it albumen tears
for my wasted sperm.

These are the nettles that prick my self-esteem.
From every cut the same question bleeds:
What have I ever done of permanence and worth?

I am a clown's bladder,
a skin balloon, a vacant bubble
drifting through the greenish flux of time,
while vague leviathans of primal fear
glide threateningly athwart my blind and fragile bows.

Now, even the cheerless, flickering vitality of dread
is ebbing in fatigue.
My chest no longer wants to push
against the suffocating weight of all
that is indifferent to my fate.
My sex no longer cares to rise
and oppose its will to that indifference.

I think the membrane cannot hold
much longer before it tears,
before I am sucked out of myself
into oblivion, like human detritus disgorging
from the ruptured fuselage of a plane.

The first stanza presented images of my life disordered and made purposeless by exhaustion. The second evoked the guilt and shame I felt for that waste. The third probed my sense of fragility and vulnerability to death. The fourth moved toward despair and my lack of will to struggle any longer. And, the fifth ended the poem with an image of the total physical and spiritual disintegration that I felt so imminent. Throughout it all, the images of hollow things collapsing, rupturing, or being pricked open specifically referenced my respiratory failure. Reading the poem over to myself after it was done, I was appalled at its morbidity. I knew the feelings described had been mine, but I almost felt as though I were reading about someone else. I realized how putting my feelings in artistic form had released me from them and helped me to appreciate the distance I had traveled since they had possessed me.

Vital as this self-healing was to my emotional recovery, it was matched, if not surpassed, in importance by Ruth's love. I had feared that the ordeal of the tracheotomy would be too steep a price for her to want to pay for being involved with me and that she would be repelled by my new mechanized body. Neither of these fears proved true. While I was in the hospital she remained connected and committed, going through the changes along with me. Her frequent visits were the happiest, most eagerly anticipated events of my days. And, when I remonstrated with her about tiring herself out and neglecting herself to spend so much time with me, she told me—as she would continue to tell me whenever I felt guilty about taking more than giving—that she was there of her own free will and because she wanted to be.

Though I felt torn by the conflicting claims of the brave adult and the rebellious child in me, Ruth accepted and loved both. She used to hold me and tell me it was okay to cry and rage. I did not have to prove myself to her. By embracing me as I was—with my tracheotomy, my fears, my confusions—she helped me feel that I was still worthwhile.

Ruth's acceptance extended as well to the mundane, tiresome demands of my physical care—the new ones like suctioning and stoma cleaning as well as all the old ones like dressing and transferring. When I got home from the hospital and we had a chance to recommence our courtship in a more natural way, she showed a marvelous ability to incorporate those demands into a pattern of our intimacy. Everything she did for me she was able to turn into a gesture of love. By doing so, she taught me not to regret my need for care and hate that aspect of myself.

Almost exactly one year after my surgery, Ruth and I were married by Jennifer. We felt a sense of continuity and completion that she, who had helped us through a difficult time, was now officially ushering us into a new era of happiness. In the ceremony, we remembered the poignant lessons of adjustment. "Only a little over a year ago I was very ill," I told our family and friends, "and the future seemed rapidly to be closing in on me. Now it has miraculously opened again. I have my health and my dear love, Ruth, to enjoy it with. The love Ruth has given me is a creative force that has transformed me and my life. I find myself bolder, more confident in work, more creative than before. At its best love seems to transform the world itself. From being a fearful, lonely place it becomes a place where I can belong."

Ruth, in her turn, reminded our guests that "a year ago, Paul was in the hospital, adjusting to life with a 'tech.' We learned to accept this extraordinary experience as part of our relationship, and not to view it as an interruption of the natural progression of our lives together. I came to understand the meaning of the 'chuppa.' Our 'chuppa'—that is, our home—is always with us, whether it be a two-bedroom apartment or one-half of a crowded hospital room."

We pledged to live together in love, sharing our joys and sorrows, and to do our best to nourish and refresh each other's spirit during our lives together. Then we ended our ceremony with the beautiful Shaker hymn, "Simple Gifts." "'Tis a gift to be simple, 'tis a gift to be free," we all sang together. Reflecting on the year just passed, I thought that, of course, life was far from simple. It was full of complicated trials and suffering. Yet, I also believed that one might be free, even so—free of despair, free to enjoy love, creativity, and all the rich panoply of sensations that constitute being alive.

Today my life is richer than it has ever been. The tracheotomy has given me back such vitality that my problem now is not lack of energy but lack of time to pursue all my interests—working, painting, writing, enjoying married life. From time to time I still envision that space-walking astronaut who symbolized my apprehensions. But now that image has been modified. Fear sometimes flickers across his face, but more often it is lit by expressions of awe and delight at the wonderful adventure he is privileged to have. Like him, my adventure, my life, goes on, and I have many more reasons to be glad than sorry.

27

VENTILATING FEELINGS

Hugh Newton-John, M.B.B.S., F.R.C.P., F.R.A.C.P.

On the door of the respiratory unit where I work is a small card which reads, "Every day the same damn thing: Breathe, breathe, breathe. . . ." How much frustration is compressed into this little jibe! We, the observers, who take our own breathing completely for granted, discover with a real sense of shock that many of our patients are aware of the effort they must expend on every breath.

Breathing is an automatic function. Most of the time, we are unaware of the process. We constantly use our breath as a tool to carry out many of our social rituals, again without so much as a second thought. We cry out in joy at the sight of an old friend. We groan at bad news. We shout at a deaf neighbor. These various sounds allow communication and the expression and release of emotions. The use of breath to produce these sounds is spontaneous, immediate, and often involuntary. Our everyday speech is full of nuance, expressing far more than the words alone, not only through alterations in timing, pitch, and volume, but also through the unconscious use of body language.

In all cultures which espouse mental and physical practices to enhance spiritual and physical well-being, breath is central. Yogic traditions and meditation practices, for example, invoke the breath as being of transcendental importance to the well-being of the individual. Pranayama, or the ancient Indian science of breath, uses sophisticated and advanced methods to control the rate, depth, and quality of the breath, in order to induce profound changes in consciousness. There are similar methods of altering awareness by using the breath in numerous eastern exercises, including Siddha Yoga, Sufi practice, Taoist meditation, and Soto Zen Buddhism. In the west, hyperventilation as a technique has only recently been used to induce beneficial and healing changes in awareness and to allow release of inner feelings (Grof, 1988).

In western culture, awareness of the inner value and importance of the breath, other than simply as a physiological function, is almost totally lacking. Indeed, in many western societies, the audible expression of feelings in public, for example by openly sobbing, is regarded in men as a sign of unmanliness and in women as a weakness. Shouting with rage or screaming with delight are regarded as the prerogatives of youth, of crowds at football matches, or of certain "ethnic" minorities. Nevertheless, we all manage to use our breath in a wide variety of ways, both subtle and gross, to help express our inner feelings and to relieve tensions. The ability to produce nothing more dramatic than a deep sigh can be most calming in times of stress. What if we were unable to perform this simple respiratory manuver because our breathing muscles are too weak? What would it be like to *be* breathed and have no control over the subtle patterns of breath we take for granted? What happens to a ventilated patient who grieves yet is unable to sob or shriek?

It might be argued that it does not matter, as nothing can be done: if you cannot breathe, you cannot breathe. Nonsense! Understanding these issues *does* matter. More and more patients with respiratory insufficiency are now being managed on ventilators. Their life expectancy is being expanded as their disability worsens. They have to learn to live in society and cope with a progressively severe disturbance of breathing. How *do* they cope? What can we learn from their experience? What do physicians need to know to help them on their journey? These are the questions.

Those who deal with newly ventilated patients realize how much time may need to be spent with them as they struggle towards a new wellness on the ventilator, a process which can take months. It is not just a matter of attaching a machine to a patient. Are there important differences at the emotional level between natural and mechanical breathing, and in the "meaning" of the breath for the ventilated person?

Patients may initially fight their ventilator as an "enemy" every step of the way; to these patients the machine seems to have great symbolic, almost mythical, significance. Others tolerate the control the ventilator has over their breathing most of the time, then may suddenly decompensate and become distressed, even panicky, the machine at that moment feeling like an unbearable intrusion. Some see the ventilator as a symbol of their slow progression to death and it is bitterly, albeit silently, resented. When they experience uncomfortable emotions they may target the ventilator as the cause and project all the anger, fear, and frustration they feel onto the machine. Thus, their choking attacks, abdominal bloating, or insomnia are too easily interpreted as the cause of their emotional distress, rather than the other way about. The physician may then collude in the process of tracking down the problem (with the ventilator, circuit, humidifier, or whatever). Unless the real cause of the symptoms is appreciated, they persist or worsen.

These general remarks preface a brief discussion of some ways a ventilator may interfere with communication and with the normal expression and release of feelings through the breath.

There are two main areas to consider:

1. *The physical presence of a ventilator,* as well as the connections between ventilator and patient, may have direct adverse social effects.

2. *The loss of certain breath modes,* preventing communication and spontaneous expressions of emotion.

THE MACHINE

The ventilator may be terrifying to a patient. An iron lung (or tank ventilator) is a huge coffin-like device with a lid which comes down with dreadful finality, leaving only the head showing. Patients become untouchable in a literal sense. They are cut off from normal intimacy and warmth, especially at night. One cannot share an iron lung! Patients who change to nose-mask ventilation after being in an iron lung for years say that the real delight is to be able to sleep with their partner again; they would never go back in "that thing" again. The experience of the lid coming down is very alarming for most, and often produces claustrophobia and a fear of never getting out. In an iron lung, a seal is needed around the neck. This is usually quite tight and can cause unpleasant choking sensations, compounding the orthopnea many ventilator-dependant patients have. The death image is constantly present because the ventilator looks like a coffin, an insistent reminder of mortality. The size of the machine is such that visitors who have not seen one before often are so appalled they cannot relate to the patient because of their own anxiety. It is not surprising that patients prefer not to be visited while they are "in the box." Normal interpersonal relationships are almost impossible when one is supine with only the face visible.

It is not only the iron lung which causes psychosocial problems. A face or nasal mask, now commonly used in patients with less severe ventilatory insufficiency, covers a surprisingly large proportion of the face and is often manufactured from colored plastic. A lumpy pink mask on the nose makes the patient look like a clown or "Miss Piggy," and interferes both with self-image and communication. The patient is embarrassed about looking silly, and the onlooker finds it hard to read the subtleties of facial expression so necessary for intimate conversation. No patient will tolerate a mask for long on his or her face during waking hours for these reasons. Loss of contact through the blocking of facial expressions is unacceptable. A mouthpiece may not seem so intrusive but may similarly make the patient unacceptable to his or her family. One patient told me that in all the family photographs in which he appeared as a child, his mouthpiece was removed when the picture was taken. A tracheostomy has some more obvious adverse effects on social normalcy. Mucus is ugly and embarrassing. There is a hole in the body which should not be there, like an extra orifice. Many patients, especially females, cover up the hole in public. The fear of being repugnant to others may take a long time to overcome. Adventures into public places with a tracheostomy may be infrequent for these reasons.

Other items of equipment, such as valves and tubing, may cause a patient social distress if ugly, bulky, or generally "industrial" to look at. The cosmetic issue is often not even considered by staff used to intensive care ventilation, where such matters are not relevant. Even the design of modern portable ventilators leaves a lot to be desired from this perspective.

LOSSES

Ventilated patients are fortunate if they need a machine to support them only at night. There are, however, many patients who have almost no reserve ventilatory function and who require breathing assistance day and night. These patients are likely to face many potential losses. It is hard for "normal breathers" to intuitively understand the implications of being ventilated, as so much of normal breath-related activity is unconscious or effortless. A number of conversations with ventilator users has helped me to more clearly understand the extent of these losses.

Speech

Most of us are unaware of the many subtleties in our speech patterns which contribute richness, humor, and meaning to our conversations. We take them for granted. A patient on a ventilator loses a great deal of this.

Punctuated speech is inevitable while on a ventilator. The smooth and spontaneous flow of words is constantly interrupted by machine breaths. The first loss is therefore *spontaneity*. Telling jokes (*silliness*) becomes difficult because timing is so critical. Witty conversation is rendered clumsy for the same reason; quick interjections work only if the timing is impeccable. There is no way to raise or lower the pitch or volume of the voice, so nuances are harder to communicate. Speech while on a ventilator is often of low volume and may be difficult to hear, adding to social problems.

Singing

It is easy for most of us to whistle or sing to relieve boredom, to celebrate well-being, or just to enjoy the emotional release the activity provides. We sing along with our favorite tunes on the radio, we bellow happily in the shower, we hum at work.

Ventilated patients would love to sing along or sing to their families, but find it very difficult for the same reasons as for speech. Rhythm and spontaneity are lost, which takes all the fun out of the process.

Sighing

People sigh frequently and often unconsciously from frustration, tiredness, pent-up distress, or just for the pleasure of it. A good sigh while on a typical home ventilator can only be simulated by turning up the machine settings, a deliberate and unspontaneous act. The lack of immediacy, as well as the physical nuisance of altering the settings on the ventilator, makes it hardly worth the effort.

Sobbing

The release of pent-up sadness or happiness through crying is for most of us a sudden and unexpected event that makes us feel better. For a patient on a ventilator, the expression of grief through "silent crying" with tears and a concomitant release of emotion is possible, but noisy sobbing is not. However, crying may be deliberately avoided by ventilated patients, because the resultant accumulation of secretions is distressing (and even dangerous, if they are unable to blow their nose or cough), and it is dauntingly unspontaneous to have to anticipate the need for help.

Screaming

A really good yell is not possible when on a ventilator. A loud noise may be possible, but because of timing and the constant interruption of breathing by the ventilator, a shout sounds contrived, so the choice is often made to avoid it.

I have focused on losses that relate to the breath. There is one more significant loss, which is due to the need for the ventilator to be ever-present: *silence*. We can, when we need peace, seek out a silent place and be still with ourselves. A person who is ventilated full-time never experiences true silence, and sudden silence has the frightening meaning that the ventilator has stopped.

Ventilated patients who were normal as children remember what they once could do, what they once had, and experience such losses as very real. What compensations are there? Close physical contact, particularly sexual contact, allows the ventilated person to experience a warm and secure release of feelings. Sexual release is a vital compensation for the restricted nature of a ventilated person's intimacy, a fact which should be more widely recognized and acknowledged. For many reasons, sex is often avoided as a topic by professionals involved with the disabled. Let us remember that it may be the main way that a ventilated person copes with "the loss of the breath."

REFERENCE

Grof, Stanislav, *The Adventure of Self-discovery* (Albany: State University of New York Press, 1988), pp. 170–184.

28

REPRESSION, REGRESSION, AND RESPIRATION

Ventilators and the Post-Polio Patient

Margaret E. Backman, Ph.D.

Many polio patients experienced respiratory problems when they contracted the disease. Today, a significant number of former patients are beginning to experience a deterioration in their condition, sometimes accompanied by pain, muscle weakness, and respiratory difficulties. The newly identified syndrome is commonly referred to as the Post-polio Syndrome, Post-polio Sequalae, or the Late Effects of Polio. With the emergence of the new symptoms comes a resurfacing of the old fears and memories that had long been repressed.

To appreciate the emotional upheavals of post-polio patients, it is important to understand how the disease and its treatment were originally experienced. This chapter takes a historical perspective, focusing on the psychological reactions to ventilators that were used during the polio epidemics of the 1950s, with particular attention to the reactions to the commonly used tank respirator or "iron lung."

WHAT IS THE POST-POLIO SYNDROME?

Estimates of the number of polio survivors in the United States range all the way from 200,000 to 1.6 million. At least 132,000 people were struck with the disease during the 1952–1954 epidemic. Now, decades later, many who felt they had overcome the illness and made their adjustments are beginning to experience increasing weakness and pain, the cause of which is yet to be fully understood (Halstead and Wiechers, 1985, 1987; Laurie, 1980; National Center for Health Statistics, U.S. Department of Health,

1987; National Institute of Handicapped Research, 1986; Roosevelt Warm Springs Institute for Rehabilitation, 1982, 1983).

From 20 to 50 percent of polio survivors over 40 years of age are reported as exhibiting these late effects; it is expected that the percentage will increase as the population ages and physicians become more astute in their diagnoses (Halstead and Wiechers, 1985, 1987; Horowitz, 1985; Laurie, 1980; Laurie, et al., 1984). A paradoxical effect of the success of the polio vaccines is that there are few physicians today who have training or experience in treating polio patients. Most health care providers are unaware of the condition, and patients, frustrated and scared, must search for help. Misdiagnosis is not uncommon.

As the extent and nature of the original disabilities vary, so do these later symptoms. Patients with even minor deformities or weakness of the spine or limb may develop painful degenerative joint disease or nerve compression as a result of continuous weight bearing on the joints from everyday activities. Weakened back muscles may result in severe scoliosis, necessitating surgery. Some who were able to walk without auxiliary devices now have to use crutches or a brace; others may need a wheelchair. Those with limited breathing reserve may need mechanical assistance.

One of the complications of poliomyelitis was acute respiratory failure. Many patients needed mechanical ventilation for months or years, either full-time or part-time, due to chronic ventilatory insufficiency. Some still must rely on ventilators for survival; others were able to give up the devices after the acute stages of the illness had passed. The more fortunate suffered no breathing difficulties and were left with little or no residual effects of the crippling disease.

With the advent of the late effects of polio, however, increasing numbers of former patients are finding that they are developing new respiratory problems, some for the first time (Bach, et al., 1987; Weiler, 1988).

ASSISTED VENTILATION DURING THE POLIO EPIDEMICS: A HISTORICAL PERSPECTIVE

The United States was not as advanced as Britain, Scandinavia, and other countries in Europe in the use of controled or automatic ventilation in the 1950s. In 1952 there was a major outbreak of poliomyelitis in Copenhagen. In reaction to this epidemic, European countries established respiratory centers throughout Europe, using various techniques for mechanically assisted respiration. Although mechanical ventilation was still in its infancy in the US, during the polio epidemics of the 1950s Bower and his associates in Los Angeles lowered the mortality rate for those with bulbar-type polio from 90 percent to 20 percent, using a technique based on "the Drinker iron lung, tracheotomy, Bennett's extra-pressure device, and high humidity" (Dobkin, 1972, p. 78). This attested to the importance of assisted mechanical respiration for polio patients with respiratory involvement. About then, the National Foundation for Infantile Paralysis organized respirator centers in various parts of the United States. The centers relied mainly on the tank respirator. It was not until the mid-1950s that researchers in the United States began developing ventilators for long-term respiratory care, and there has been great progress in the devices since then, especially with the introduction of portable ventilators.

The eventual development of the Salk and Sabin vaccines and the mass inoculations that followed led to the eradication of polio in the United States, Canada, and Europe. However, many patients still must rely on ventilators. Fortunately, the techniques available, including portable ventilators, are more sophisticated and less restrictive than those available 40 years ago. As the incidence of the disease declined, the polio centers were closed, and the National Foundation for Infantile Paralysis focused its attention on other areas, dropping reference to infantile paralysis (as polio was then called) from its name. With the shift of emphasis went the training and resulting expertise in treating this disease. Thus, when former patients began developing symptoms decades later, there were few practicing physicians who had the needed expertise. Many patients with post-polio symptoms were misdiagnosed, or the symptoms were minimized or ignored, since the disease no longer readily came to mind.

THE ROLE OF THE VENTILATOR IN THE PSYCHOLOGICAL ADJUSTMENT OF PATIENTS WITH POST-POLIO SYMPTOMS

To understand what post-polio patients may be going through emotionally now, it is important to understand how they reacted psychologically when they first contracted the disease (Backman, 1987, 1989). As new physical symptoms emerge, psychological issues with ties to the past begin to surface as well.

The patients' premorbid personalities played important roles in the way they reacted to the initial bout with polio. Those who had a fear of failure, for example, would be devastated by the inability to take care of themselves and would become particularly concerned about the future. Those subject to depression would become more depressed. Those with obsessive-compulsive personalities would be concerned about every detail of their care and their body functions in an attempt to gain some kind of control. Those already struggling with issues of dependency would be particularly upset when becoming dependent upon a ventilator.

The Threat of Death

When the muscles of respiration are paralyzed, the inability to breathe and the feeling of suffocation are a direct attack upon the ego. The possibility of death is very real.

The fear of death during the acute phase of polio was so overwhelming that patients handled it through *massive repression* (repression so extensive that it pushes unwanted memories from conscious memory, taking with it associated thoughts and feelings as well). Today many post-polio patients may have no awareness of what happened to them, or only vague or partial memories. Yet the thought that they may have to go through the experience again awakens powerful emotions that are bewildering and frightening. After the acute phase, death by asphyxiation was rare, but the sense of threat nevertheless remained. Fear of death was revealed by patients' concerns about mechanical or electrical failure of the respiratory equipment. As patients increased unassisted breathing time, there was a notable decrease in anxieties. However, fear of death associated with the acute phase of polio was often transferred onto the mechanical device, a tangible object onto which patients could project their more existential fears.

Psychological concerns with asphyxiation were associated with the mask, which was sometimes used to assist in ventilation. The mask may have been used, for example, when a patient was being moved and was temporarily out of the "iron lung." Later in life, patients may have panic attacks when their faces are covered or when they develop shortness of breath under stress.

The Psychological Meaning of the Respirator

The respirator became important to polio patients, since it saved their lives. Patients developed different attachments to the machines, which were loved and hated at the same time. On one hand, the tank respirator offered a sense of security. It became a substitute body or "a womblike structure which the patient [feared] to leave" (Glud and Blane, 1956). This psychological attachment made it harder for patients to be weaned from the respirator, particulary since their bodies were so changed, having become being weak and barely functional. Yet there was anger, too, as patients hated the dependency and loss of control that the respirator signified.

Psychological Dependency

Most polio deaths were from paralysis of the patients' respiratory area. Thus, the ventilation devices gave patients "the breath of life." H.E. Van Riper, Medical Director for the National Foundation for Infantile Paralysis, reports seeing patients in iron lungs who had "almost forgotten how to breathe for themselves" (1956, p. 45)—a condition which often continued long after the muscles were capable of providing adequate ventilation of the lungs.

Patients had to be psychologically weaned from iron lungs and other respiratory aides. As a result of this dependent state, many patients returned home lacking in confidence and experiencing difficulty with the ordinary activities of daily living. Over time, through the step-by-step process of rehabilitation and encouragement from family and friends, patients gradually regained both the physical and psychological strength to move ahead.

Restrictions in the Life Space and Psycho-Social Deprivation

There is a psychological deprivation associated with respirators, particularly the iron lung. Patients cannot be stroked or held; the comfort that comes from touching is denied them (Report of the Surgeon General's Workshop, 1982).

When in the tank respirator, there is a sense of being an "island unto themselves" with little communication. If there was a dome over their head while they were in the tank respirator, it was difficult to be heard, cutting them off even more from their environment. Another factor contributing to the restrictions in communication was the loss of the use of the hands, which are used to feed, dress, and communicate, both in writing and by expressive gestures. Patients learned to use other people as extensions of themselves.

Not only did patients have to contend with paralysis, but being dependent upon a ventilator severely limited their mobility. Such limitations are hard at any age, but for young growing patients it was particularly difficult. Movement is one way individuals discharge energy and tension. When movement is thwarted, frustration, both physical and psychological, mounts.

The lack of mobility the patients suffered limited them physiologically, in terms of taking care of their oral, genital, and excretory needs. They would feel shame, embarrassment, and anger. Patients who could not take care of these very basic matters felt denied and angered at their dependency.

Polio patients on ventilators often spent months in the hospital, not knowing the difference between night and day. Only hospital rituals helped to keep them organized and aware. Small changes in a patient's environment, such as the position of the bed or a change of roommates, could be disturbing. A stable environment signifies security, and small changes can take on enormous significance when space is restricted.

The overhead mirror used with tank respirators helped patients to see beyond their limited environment, but what was seen was portions of people's bodies and portions of the area beyond. Thus, not only was self-perception fragmented, but the perception of others and the outside world was disjointed.

Self-Concept and Integrity

By "self-image" we refer to the picture of our self and our body that we have in our mind. The picture develops over time and begins to form by nine months of age. It is representative of the present and the past and changes as the individual learns new skills and has new experiences. For those in an "iron lung," self-image is challenged on a very basic level. Patients become overly concerned with "their head and its functions; with excretory functions; with genital functions . . ." (Glud and Blane, 1956, p. 30).

The emphasis on the head is reinforced by the use of the overhead mirror. Prugh and Tagiuri (1954) reported that those who used an overhead mirror while in the tank respirator viewed themselves as "heads," with the head being disproportionately large in contrast to the body (which was hidden by the tank). Most give-and-take behaviors centered around the mouth, which was seen as the most prominent part of the head and the one area of control that the patient had. The mouth was also the main source of communication and satisfaction. Even sexual gratification could be achieved through the head and the mouth, with patients telling sexual jokes (to relieve sexual tension) or feeling sensual pleasure when stroked on the head and face—something not always appreciated by those not so immobilized.

Patients reported feeling different from others as a result of their experiences. Although the most psychological meanings were associated with the "iron lung," the other mechanical breathing devices also became part of the new and often distorted self-images. For example, children who used a chest respirator (a plastic cuirass) often referred to themselves as "Space Men," revealing that they sensed that they looked different or odd.

Over time, the image that patients had of themselves was shattered. The idea of being an "athlete," a "bread-winner," or a "housewife" had been altered. Thoughts of being strong, pretty, or invincible no longer had any meaning. Many patients became depressed as they began to feel that they could no longer live up to their aspirations.

The sense of the body's integrity and what psychoanalysts call primary narcissism were also challenged by dependency on mechanical breathing devices. People usually think things happen to others, not to them. With the attack of polio, this sense of invulnerability was shattered.

Body image was also affected if the patient needed to have a tracheotomy to help with breathing. There may have been concerns about the future, coupled with unrealistic hopes. Suppression or denial of the effect of the procedure on the patient's body often lead to overt anxiety and further depression. The feelings of mutilation could result in personality changes, if not worked through in counseling or therapy.

Threats to the body's integrity were also associated with fears of annihilation. This could lead to *regression* in behavior and evidence of the psychological defense called *depersonalization*, e.g., the feeling that the body or parts of the body are not part of the self. Patients felt that they were outside of their bodies, looking at themselves, watching what was happening, feeling that it was not happening to them. The feelings of depersonalization or dissociation, which may have occurred during the acute phase of polio, and particularly when suffering respiratory insufficiency in the iron lung, may reappear years later—perhaps when a patient has to undergo surgery and is given an anesthetic, or if he or she needs mechanical assistance for breathing again. Even the thought of needing assisted ventilation for the post-polio symptoms could trigger feelings of depersonalization. Patients may fear they are going "crazy" when experiencing these feelings, and those treating them, not considering the patient's previous history, may unfortunately agree, not realizing the psychological basis for the behavior.

Mental Status Changes

The acute phase of polio left patients feeling "helpless, confused, often near panic, with bizarre physical and psychic experiences" (Glud and Blane, 1956, p. 28). Many emerged from the upheaval to find themselves dependent upon mechanical aid for respiration, and usually completely quadraplegic.

During the acute phase, attacks on the respiratory system resulted in psychological disturbances for many patients. Glud and Blane described this as organic clouding of the sensorium, contributed to by hypoventilation with carbon dioxide retention. This reduced the control of higher cortical centers and resulted in periods of hyperactivity, vagueness, disorientation, anxiety, and/or dream productions, which patients often could not distinguish from reality. Partial or complete amnesia of the acute stage was not uncommon. Patients not properly prepared for being placed in a tank respirator became overwhelmed with panic or completely disorganized.

Post-polio patients may wonder why they have lapses of memory for many segments of their early treatment. Memories they do have of mental confusion make them fearful that they were crazy or had been hallucinating. In the early years of working with patients on ventilators, there were not enough trained psychologists or other mental health professionals available to help patients deal psychologically with the many adjustments they had to make.

STAGES OF PSYCHOLOGICAL DEVELOPMENT: THE CHILD AND POLIO

Most of those who contracted polio were children. How they experienced the disease, including the inability to breath and assisted ventilation, was determined in large part by their developmental age (Backman, 1989). Many were only infants or small children who have only the barest memory of the experience. The illness may have occurred at the preverbal stage of development, when they did not have language to help them express their feelings. Memories of the events associated with polio were stored in their unconscious without verbal labels, making it hard to retrieve them. However, the feelings associated with the stored memories can be triggered at a later date, leaving the person bewildered and confused by the emerging emotions or behavior that seem to come from nowhere. Former patients, for example, may experience isolated symptoms such as free-floating anxiety or shortness of breath in stressful situations later in life. Without psychotherapy, they may not realize why they are experiencing these feelings and may find themselves in a state of panic, thinking that something is wrong with them mentally.

Theoretically, if they had polio when they were older than three years of age, when the verbal and cognitive functions were more mature, they would most likely develop more complex neurotic patterns as a result of the illness, rather than the isolated symptoms infants would develop. Later in life, the neurotic patterns would appear as unresolved issues of dependency, submission, and helplessness—problems which become more intense as they experience the frightening post-polio symptoms.

After the age of three, when children are becoming more aware of their bodies and have fearful fantasies, even seeing another child needing assistance for breathing can be terrifying. They may interpret the assault on the body as a punishment.

Typically, children do not comprehend the realities of death until they are about eight to ten years of age. However, those who have had to depend upon machines to breathe may realize much earlier the possibility of their own death—even before they are psychologically ready to handle this. Those who did not have respiratory difficulties may have seen others using ventilators, some of whom may have died. Thus, the fear of death becomes a reality that gets repressed with other frightening memories.

The traumatic experience of not being in charge of something as basic as one's own breathing would interact with the usual developmental issues a child struggles with at various ages. Very young children may not understand why their parents cannot help them. Older children may feel abandoned, leaving them frightened and mistrustful of their parents and authority figures in general.

The child who must go through long-term hospitalization is cut off from the usual experiences of childhood. This is true for any hospitalized child, but the effects are especially noticeable when the child's mobility and self-perception are determined by a mechanical device such as a ventilator (Seidenfeld, 1956). Children in hospitals and convalescent homes often do not have regular schooling and fall behind, academically and socially. Reentry into school is difficult and embarrassing. The children may be mature and immature at the same time. Not being able to socialize with peers left many socially awkward when they were later respirator-free and living at home. Yet, having spent so much time with adults in the hospitals and respiratory centers, they revealed a maturity that others their age did not have and could not understand. Thus, when they returned home, they felt they no longer fit in.

For the adolescent, lack of control and dependency can be particularly devastating. This is a stage when young people learn to separate from their parents and take control of their lives and bodies. Having polio would be traumatic enough, but becoming dependent upon a machine to breathe often leads to a psychological regression that carries over when the adolescent is back home and off the ventilator, taking the form of rebellious acting out or the contrary, overdependency and anger.

THE LATE EFFECTS OF POLIO IN THE '90s: PSYCHOLOGICAL ISSUES

Although many former polio patients are now adults, their early experiences with polio still play a role in their lives. In most cases, the unpleasant memories have been forced back into their unconscious and the individuals have gone on with their lives. Under stressful circumstances, when the late effects of polio begin to appear, the disturbing feelings surface as well. "I thought I had put this all behind me," one former polio patient cried.

Not only are physical symptoms returning now, but patients are having to deal again with doctors and hospitals and clinics. This time it is different. They are not as naive or as uninformed as before. They have the frightening memories and face the uncertain future they thought they had escaped. They worry about what treatments lie in wait, with mental images of ventilators fresh in their minds.

Patients' reactions may seem extreme and inappropriate, unless there is an awareness of the unresolved issues that have been repressed. When patients find themselves becoming weaker and unable to do many of the things they used to do, they naturally become afraid. Those who sense new difficulties with breathing wonder how much more deterioration will occur, will this be progressive, or will the process plateau? They wonder how long it will take and what lies in store for them for the future. It is not like having the disease the first time. Now they are older, understand more, and have already lived through the terror of the original bout with polio.

CAUTIONS TO PHYSICIANS

The behavior that the physicians and families of post-polio patients see today is often regressive, e.g., resisting medical advice, taking risks, not going for tests, smoking, and asking endless questions. Yet this behavior can be seen as an attempt to gain control over uncontrollable feelings and events—a fear that includes for some the possibility of becoming ventilator-dependent after years of being ventilator-free. For others, who have been ventilator-dependent for many years, there is the fear of losing what respiratory function they have and facing uncertain death. Some cautions are in order when working with such patients:

1. Do not jump to conclusions about patients' difficult behavior. Although patients' reactions to their decreased breathing capacity may seem extreme, keep in mind their earlier experiences with polio, and be aware that patients may be emotionally reliving feelings from the past, in addition to making adjustments in the present.
2. Do not assume because new improved ventilation devices are available that patients will accept them easily. Memories from the past will set up resistances, at least initially.
3. Do not make the mistake of saying to patients, "Well, you've been on a ventilator before, so this is nothing new to you." Do not assume that familiarity lessens anxiety; on the contrary, it often enhances it.
4. Do not jump to conclusions about patients' noncompliance, argumentativeness, or other difficult behavior. Part of this is fear, part is resistance to becoming dependent again. A large part is a lack of trust in the medical profession, a profession that previously encouraged polio patients to push themselves, to excel, and now tells them that they may have worn themselves out by doing too much. No wonder post-polio patients question authority and are hesitant to follow medical advice. They question whether today's post-polio specialists know what they are doing, and many former polio patients do not even seek medical help, not wanting to get involved with the medical world again, hoping their illness will stabilize.
5. Use mental health professionals as part of the treatment team. Patients may need to go through these emotional upheavals in order to work through unresolved issues and regain control of their feelings. Although going back on a ventilator is not a pleasant prospect, the extreme fear and depression can be made more manageable if patients have the assistance of trained mental health professionals.

REFERENCES

Bach, J.R., A.S. Alba, E. Bodofsky, F.J. Curran, and M. Schultheiss, "Glossopharyngeal Breathing and Noninvasive Aids in the Management of the

Post-polio Respiratory Insufficiency," in L.S. Halstead and D.O. Wiechers, eds., *Research and Clinical Aspects of the Late Effects of Poliomyelitis* (Miami: Symposia Foundation, 1987), pp. 99–113.

Backman, M.E., "The Post-polio Patient: Psychological Issues," *Journal of Rehabilitation* 1987, 53(4): 23–26.

Backman, M.E., *The Psychology of the Physically Ill Patient: A Clinician's Guide* (New York: Plenum Press, 1989).

Dobkin, A.B., *Ventilators and Inhalation Therapy*, 2nd ed. (Boston: Little, Brown, 1972).

Glud, E., and H.T. Blane, "Body Image Changes in Patients with Respiratory Poliomyelitis, *The Nervous Child* 1956, 11(2): 25–39.

Halstead, L., and D. Wiechers, eds., *Late Effects of Poliomyelitis* (Miami: Symposia Foundation, 1985).

Halstead, L., and D. Wiechers, eds., *Research and Clinical Aspects of the Late Effects of Polio Myelitis* (Miami: Symposia Foundation, 1987).

Horowitz, J., "Polio's Painful Legacy," *New York Times Sunday Magazine* (July 7, 1985): 16–23.

Laurie, G., ed., "Respiratory Rehabilitation and Post-polio Aging Problems," *Rehabilitation Gazette* 1980, 23: 3–10.

Laurie, G., F. Maynard, D. Fischer, and J. Raymond, eds., *Handbook on the Late Effects of Poliomyelitis for Physicians and Survivors* (St. Louis, MO: Gazette International Networking Institute, 1984).

National Center for Health Statistics, *National Health Interview Survey* (Washington, DC: U.S. Department of Health, 1987).

National Institute of Handicapped Research, *The Late Effects of Poliomyelitis*, Office of Special Education and Rehabilitation Services, Rehabilitation Brief ISSN: 0732-2623. 9(9) (Falls Church, VA: PSI International, 1986).

Prugh, D., and C. Tagiuri, "Emotional Aspects of the Respirator Care of Patients with Poliomyelitis," *Psychosomatic Medicine* 1954, 16: 104–128.

Roosevelt Warm Springs Institute for Rehabilitation, Warm Springs, Georgia, *Polio News* 1982, 1(1): 2–5.

Roosevelt Warm Springs Institute for Rehabilitation, Warm Springs, Georgia, *Polio News* 1983, 1(2): 2–4.

Seidenfeld, M.A., "Polio and Personality," *The Nervous Child* 1956, 11(2): 6–9.

US Department of Health and Human Services, *Report of the Surgeon General's Workshop on Children with Handicaps and Their Families. Case example: The Ventilator-dependent Child* (Washington, DC: DHHS publication # phs-83-50194, 1982).

Van Riper, H. E., "The Parent of the Polio Child," *The Nervous Child* 1956, 11(2): 40–47.

Weiler, R.L., "Underventilation: A Warning," *Polio Network News* Spring 1988, 4(2): 1–3.

29

REGIONAL HOME CARE PROGRAM FOR VENTILATOR-DEPENDENT PATIENTS

Report of the First Five Years

Edward Anthony Oppenheimer, M.D.

INTRODUCTION

A seven-year Regional Pilot Project was started in November 1985, to enable long-term ventilator-dependent (LTVD) patients to be discharged to home care, from nine Kaiser Foundation Hospitals (KFH) in Southern California. This was a health services research and demonstration project. Prior to 1985 there was no organized experience with home mechanical ventilation (HMV) at these hospitals, and stable highly dependent LTVD patients sometimes occupied intensive care unit (ICU) beds for years. During the seven-year project a total of 91 hospital-trapped LTVD children and adults were transferred to care at home with their families. The quality of care (QC) at home was found to be similar to hospital, and the quality of life (QL) improved. KFH acute care bed utilization and program cost effectiveness were improved. This initial report covers the first five years, the first 60 patients.

These patients were previously "hospital trapped": medically stable long-term tracheostomy ventilator-dependent patients who remained in acute care hospitals (usually intensive care units). Most were survivors of unexpected admission for intensive care. The patients were severely disabled and required assistance with all or most activities of daily living and self-care. There is usually little "free time" off the ventilator. The patient or family caregivers were able to direct the needed care, after training. Hospital discharge has not been possible because: home care equipment and supply costs are high; family and friends were unable to provide the number of hours of care required; other discharge options (e.g.: skilled nursing facilities) were not available nore acceptable; and the professional staff had little experience with high-tech home care: HMV.

OBJECTIVES

[1] To enable LTVD children and adults to have a more "normal" life at home with their ramilies and friends. [2] To relieve inappropriate KFH acute bed occupancy, and to evaluate the impact of KFH average daily bed census (ADC) and length of stay (LOS). [3] To provide a formal mechanism to provide durable medical equipment (DME) and in-home paid shift care (LVN), when needed, to support home care for KFH hospital-trapped LTVD patients. [4] To provide actual clinical and cost experience with home care compared to KFH hospital care for these ventilator-dependent Health Plan members. To incllude outcome evaluation, including QC and QL. [5] To develop, manage and evaluate a formal home care protocol, policies and procedure for LTVD patients at Kaiser Permanente medical centers throughout the Southern California region.

SUMMARY OF RESULTS

A careful HMV program was developed for selection, predischarge training, and home care support. Sixty patients were discharged to home care during the first five years of the seven-year project. Seven (11.6%) were children. 53 (88.3%) were adults. Age ranged: 1 to 81. This decreased to expected LTVD pt. average daily census for the region by over 90%. This relieved ICU beds where 63% of LTVD patients received care at KFHs, and resulted in savings in facilities costs, scarce nursing and respiratory therapist staff resources and outside costs. Home care costs averaged $344 per day (ranged from: $38 to $561 per day.) 87% of home care costs were for licensed vocational nurses (LVN) in-home nursing shift care to relive trained family caregivers. In-home paid care averaged 13.4 hours per day (range: 0 to 16). 74% need 16 hours per day LVN care when 24 hour per day ventilator-dependent. Average LVN home care costs were $24 per hour. Hourly LVN agency charges continue to increase at about 10% each year. Quality of Care (QC) was similar at home to hospital. Patients were quite stable at home.There was an average of four hospital days per year per patient. 68% required no hospital days. Overall survival at home exceeds that in published reports (particularily for patients with COPD and ALS). Quality of Life (QL) was significantly better at home. Despite severe and often progressive impairments, patients assessed their QL as better at home. For children, development is more normal; they can participate in schools and social activities. Significant family stress and burden is a continuing concern.

VENTILATOR HOME CARE SURVIVAL DATA

	1 Year	2 Year
Neuromuscular	80%	74%
Kyphoscoliosis	100%	100%
COPD	62%	54%
Malignancy	0%	0%
Interstitial	0%	0%

SIXTY PATIENTS: 1985–1990

Spinal Cord Injury	3
Kyphoscoliosis	2
ALS	8
Muscular Dystrophy	6
COPD	21
Anoxic Brain Injury	5
Other Etiologies*	7
Other Neuromuscular	8

**Other Etiologies:*	
Interstitial Lung Disease	2
CVA	1
Bronchiectasis	1
Bronchopulmonary Dysplasia	1
Malignancy	2

QUALITY OF LIFE : HOME VERSUS HOSPITAL

	Equal or Better at Home
Quality of Life at home	97%
Time with family and friends	86%
Hopeful, happy, cheerful at home	73%
Feel healthier at home	75%
Sicker at home (compared to hospital)	0%
Satisfaction with life at home	74%

QUALITY OF LIFE

Feeling of Health	
Feel healthier at home than in the hospital	75%
Feel as healthy at home as in the hospital	25%
(No one felt sicker at home than in the hospital)	

Over-all Self-assessment at Home

Feel healthy	51%
Feel sick	21%
Feel neither	27%

Feel satisfied with life at home (Despite medical problems)	74%
Often feel disatisfied with life at home:	26%
Over-all Assessment	
More satisfied with life at home than hospital	73%
Home is just as satisfactory as hospital	24%
Hospital better than home:	only 1 patient
Amount of Time with Family or Friends	
Satisfied with this at home	86%
Dissatisfied with this at home	14%
Home is more satisfactory than in hospital	72%
Better in hospital	11%

General Emotional Level: Home Vs Hospital

	Happy	Hopeful	Cheerful	Total
At Home:	20%	33%	20%	73%
In Hospital:	6%	26%	11%	43%

	Depressed	Worried	Bored	Total
At Home:	13%	3%	0%	26%
In Hospital:	29%	14%	11%	57%

One patient reported feeling sad in the hospital (none did at home). More than twice as many felt depressed in the hospital. Many were bored in the hospital, but no one felt bored at home. More than three times as many felt happy at home than in the hospital Almost twice as many were cheerful at home. Many noted varying feelings at different times of the day or week. Data from standardized questionaires.

QUALITY OF CARE

Satisfaction with Ventilator Care at Home: 100%

Ability to Handle a Medical Emergency Involving the Ventilator: Family member can do this very well: 98%

Ventilator Care at Home as Equal or Better Than Hospital: 98%

Better at home	65%
Same as at hospital	33%
Very good at home	50%
Quite good at home	45%

Worry About the Ventilator Care at Home Compared to Hospital:

Don't worry at all	72%
Worry sometimes	26%
Worry a lot:	2%

Most Common Concern Expressed: Concern about the ability of a new or a fill-in nurse.

Patient or Family Feels Able to Train New Nurses in Care Skills Needed: 86%

Family Member Feels Able to Give Care as Well or Better Than the Nurse: 96%

Satisfaction with Home Health R.N. Staff: 100%

Quality of Care: Home Versus Hospital

	Equal or Better
Over-all ventilator care at home	98%
Emergencies in ventilator care at home	98%
Little or no worry about care at home	72%
Feel able to instruct nurses in home	86%
Feel able to give care better or equal to nurse	96%

Typical Comments by Patients:
Greater comfort at home. Greater ability to socialize. Allows control over life again. Improves family life. Home is living in a "well" rather than a "sick" environment.
Data from standardized questionaires.

FOLLOW-UP WITH FAMILIES AFTER THE DEATH OF PILOT PROJECT PATIENT

Was Extension of Life Provided by Ventilator Worthwhile? Yes: 100%
Comments—Very important time for family to be together. Ventilator provided stability and reassurance. Ventilator relieved dyspnea and was no burden. Able to be

there for birth of grandchild. When mental status deteriorated it was no longer good.

Is Being at Home on a Ventilator a Good Thing to Do? Yes: 100%
Comments—Very happy at home. Able to achieve closure with this additional time. Didn't want to die in the hospital.

Would You Do It Again? Yes: 100%

What Was the Best Part?
Having husband/wife at home.
Being together and being able to help.
It was best for "mom," she was in a familiar environment.
Being at home and happy; caregivers available and timely.
Being able to continue with life, with comfort and dignity.

What Was the Hardest or Worst Part?
Nursing skills were worisome at first, then became easy.
Lack of expected nurses interfered with rest of life and work.
Not knowing whether nurses would show up. Oxygen delivery was often at the last minute.
Fear of doing the wrong thing or of equipment failure.

What Was the Impact on Your Life (family Caregiver):
Career and personal life was put on "hold."
It was good for everyone.
Better than in the hospital.

Were You Prepared and Able to Deal With Death When It Came?
Prepared and able to deal with it: 75%
Unprepared but able to deal with it: 25%

Advanced Directives—Wishes Known? Yes: 86%

Limited care desired:	57%
Wanted "everything done":	29%
Only vague information:	14%

Did You Need More Preparation for the Death? No: 100%

If This Had Been Your Problem, Would You Have Used a Ventilator?

Yes:	50%
No:	50%

Frequent comment: "I might change mind to yes if in respiratory distress."

Should Prolonging Life with Mechanical Ventilation Be an Option Available for Those Who Want to Try It? Yes: 100%

Was Stopping the Ventilator Seriously Considered at Times?

Yes: 30%
No: 70%

Would You Have Wanted to Have Ventilator Care at Home ff It Only Lasted a Month?
Yes: 100%

Most Stressful and Burdensome Aspects of Ventilator Care at Home:

Problems with LVN caregivers—availability:	45%
Anxiety and responsibility:	29%
Watching mental and physical deterioration:	5%
Loss of personal time:	10%
Financial burdens:	5%

Feeling About the Ventilator:

Helpful friend:	72%
Entrapment aspects:	28%
Threat:	0%

Helpful Personal Support Resources:

Family:	70%
Church:	35%
Friends	25%

Place of Death:

Home:	40%
Hospital:	60%

Many died at the hospital just a few hours after arriving from home.

Preferred Place of Death:

Home:	28%
Hospital:	72%

Sometimes patient preferred home more than family.

Bereavement Support:

Home Health Agency:	100%
Church group:	15%
Other	15%

Would Home Care Have Been Possible Without Pilot Project?
No: 70%
"Only with great difficulty and loss of assets": 30%

Data from a regional pilot project of the Southern California Kaiser Permanente Medical Care Program supports home care for ventilator-dependent children and adults. This health care research and demonstration project started in November 1985.

Sixty "hospital trapped" long-term ventilator-dependent (LTVD) patients were discharged home from ten Kaiser Foundation Hospitals in a coordinated program, with clearly defined process and standards. Ages ranged from 1 to 84. Comparative data is also available for 30 LTVD patients who were not "hospital trapped." The pilot project LTVD patients receive assistance with equipment, supplies, paid caregivers, and Kaiser Home Health Agency supervision and care coordination. A multi-disciplinary team provided hospital evaluation, teaching, and preparation for discharge, and coordinated home care; this included psychiatry and medical social workers.

One year survival for the pilot project LTVD patients varied: 80-100% for neuromuscular and musculoskeletal disorders; 62% for chronic obstructive lung diseases (COPD); and 0% for interstitial lung diseases or malignancy.

People who electively initiate ventilator support are usually at a higher functional level and more independent. They and their family members are able to adjust more easily. Usually 6 to 12 hours of ventilator support per day are needed initially. Home care is easily arranged. The cost of equipment and supplies can generally be arranged with available personal or community resources. Paid caregivers for shift care are not often needed. However, for many reasons, people with progressing respiratory impairment frequently avoid considering elective ventilator support.

The pilot project patients represent people whose ventilator support was initiated nonelectively with a life-threatening hospitalization and ICU care. They are more often 16- to 24-hour ventilator-dependent; more often at a low functional level and more dependent on others. Home care may be difficult to arrange. In the past many remained hospital trapped. Satisfactory home care requires two trained family members plus paid caregivers, and equipment and supplies. Costs are often beyond the capabilities of personal and community resources. However, care costs are usually lower at home than in a hospital or nursing home. The family burden is large, and community resources to support them are not well developed or funded.

Twenty (33%) of the pilot project home care patients died at home or the hospital, without evidence of adverse medical care problems. Only one pilot project COPD patient elected withdrawal of life support. This was done with support from his family and the hospital staff.

Almost all hospitalized LTVD patients who have family members to assist them are able to be successfully discharged home with this pilot project. With good medical care and social support, these patients are almost always satisfied with their quality of life, compared to the alternatives. When experienced centers arrange home care, *quality of care* is similar to hospital care, and patients assess *quality of life* at home as better than in the hospital.

REFERENCES

Baldwin-Myers, A. and E.A. Oppenheimer (1996). "Quality of life and quality of care data from a 7-year pilot project for home mechanical ventilator patients." *J Ambulatory Care Management* 19(1): 46–59.

Feldman, J. and P.G. Tuteur (1982). "Mechanical ventilation: From hospital intensive care to home." *Heart Lung* 11(2): 162–5.

Fischer, D.A. and W.S. Prentice (1982). "Feasibility of home care for certain respiratory-dependent restrictive or obstructive lung disease patients." *Chest* 82(6): 739–43.

Goldbert, A.I., A.A. Alba, E.A. Oppenheimer, and E. Roberts (1990). "Personal care attendants for people using mechanical ventilation at home." *Chest* 98: 1543.

Kinnear, W.J. and J.M. Shneerson (1985). "Assisted ventilation at home: Is it worth considering?" *Br J Dis Chest* 79(4): 313–51.

Make, B.J. and M.E. Gilmartin (1986). "Rehabilitation and home care for ventilator-assisted individuals." *Clin Chest Med* 7(4): 679–91.

Make, B.J. and M.E. Gilmartin (1990). "Mechanical ventilation in the home." *Crit Care Clin* 6(3): 785–96.

O'Donohue, W.J., Jr., R.M. Giovannoni, et al. (1986). "Long-term mechanical ventilation. Guidelines for management in the home and at alternate community sites. Report of the Ad Hoc Committee, Respiratory Care Section, American College of Chest Physicians." *Chest* 90(1 Suppl): 1S-37S.

Oppenheimer, E.A. (April 1988). "Regional Pilot Project: Home Care for Hospitalized Ventilator-Dependent Patients 1985–1987" (testimony presented to the HCFA Task Force, March 5, 1985) in: Fostering Home and Community-Based Care for Technology-Dependent Children, HCFA Publ. No. 88-02171-pp. 376–385.

Oppenheimer, E.A. (1990). "Mechanical Respiratory Support at Home." *West J Med* 153: 74.

Oppenheimer, E.A. and A.S. Baldwin-Myers (1989). "Home Care Project for Ventilator-Dependent Patients." (Abstract) *Amer Rev Resp Diseases* 139 (No. 4 part 2): A541.

Oppenheimer, E.A. and R. Essink (1987). "Home care pilot project for ventilator-dependent patients." Presented at the 53rd Annual Scientific Assembly of the American College of Chest Physicians, October 1987. (Abstract) *Chest* 92: 108S.

Ordonneau, J., E. Chailleux, et al. (1986). "Actuarial survival rate in 99 tracheostomized patients with chronic pulmonary insufficiency treated by pulmonary mechanical ventilation at home." *Eur J Respir Dis Suppl* 146: 383–8.

Peters, S.G., and R.W. Viggiano (1988). "Home mechanical ventilation." *Mayo Clin Proc* 63(12): 1208–13.

Plummer, A.L., W.J. O'Donohue, Jr., et al. (1989). "Consensus conference on problems in home mechanical ventilation." *Am Rev Respir Dis* 140(2): 555–60.

Rosen, R.L., and R.C. Bone (1988). "Economics of mechanical ventilation." *Clin Chest Med* 9(1): 163–9.

Splaingard, M.L., R.C. Frates, Jr., et al. (1983). "Home positive-pressure ventilation. Twenty years' experience." *Chest* 84(4): 376–82.

Votava, K.M., T. Cleveland, et al. (1985). "Home care of the patient dependent on mechanical ventilation: home care policy development and goal setting using outcome criteria for quality assurance." *Home Healthc Nurse* 3(2): 18–25.

30

OCCUPATIONAL THERAPY AND THE VENTILATOR-DEPENDENT PATIENT

The Impact on Psychosocial and Motoric Aspects of Activities of Daily Living

Ann Burkhardt, M.A., O.T.R.

From the time we are born and throughout our lives, growth seems to be correlated with independence. There is a lifetime struggle to escape dependence or a dependent role. Yet, when disease enters our lives we are forced to face the issue of dependency.

Chronic diseases, especially those requiring external hardware, add to the burden because they present blatant, visual clues to the public. Most individuals are content to be a face in the crowd. If external hardware must be relied upon, such individuals stand out from the crowd.

Occupational therapists work to improve or restore the ability of chronic sufferers to engage in the activities of daily living (ADLs). ADLs include basic self-care skills (grooming, washing, dressing, feeding, toileting), life management skills (household tasks, basic personal financial management tasks, use of leisure time, etc.), and job performance skills (manual dexterity, level of cognitive function to complete task ability demands, work behavior). When chronic disease impacts on one's life, all these aspects of living are involved.

Dependence, with accompanying loss of control over oneself and one's environment, surely impacts on self-esteem. The art of occupational therapy lies in the ability to teach individuals to change their style or method of doing their daily activities or to adapt the elements of those activities so that the individual regains some control in his or her life. Success with these adapted devices and techniques has the potential to enhance self-esteem and foster coping mechanisms.

Being out of breath severely limits the ability to tolerate activity. Dependence on a ventilator can so overwhelm a person that he or she may stop challenging themselves. The role of the occupational therapist is to refocus the person on achievable goals and to teach strategies for overcoming the obstacles encountered. Usually this involves relearning to live life at a pace. Timing becomes of the utmost importance.

New Yorkers live life at a thunderous pace, so perhaps this element of treatment is most poignant for them. Consider how long it takes to get washed and dressed, to eat breakfast, and to get to work. Thirty minutes to an hour may be a reasonable estimate. For a ventilator-dependent person, this may take three to four hours. Each activity may require five- to ten-minute rest intervals before the task is completed.

Being a participant in a treatment program seems overwhelming, if you consider the energy and effort required when the individual is constantly out of breath or connected to a machine.

It is, fortunately, possible for the patient to often increase endurance by pacing and repeating the sequence of activities on a daily basis, over time (weeks, months, years). Careful preparation and counseling about lost functioning may also be a factor when palliation is the goal.

I have personal experience with two situations involving ventilator-dependent persons close to me, one a relative, one a friend.

My uncle died in 1986. He had Amyotrophic Lateral Sclerosis (ALS). His form of the disease involved the bulbar functions. Basically, he could not make facial expressions, lost mouth/oral motor control, and began to experience vocal cord paralysis. In addition, his proximal muscles became weak. He could not lift his arms over his head or cut his food sitting down. He had problems standing up from low surfaces.

Many health professionals become pivotal resource people for relatives when they become ill. This was my role in my uncle's illness. Uncle Don was a chemical engineer. He was a private consultant who practiced internationally, a gardener, a sailor, a father to two men, a husband, and a grandfather. He loved dinner theater and ballroom dancing. He was sharp and bright. He loved a good argument as well as the next man, and he loved languages.

Uncle Don's disease evolved rapidly. Within four months of diagnosis he had problems putting his shirt on. Within six months, he developed dysphagia. Within nine months, he had nearly complete vocal cord paralysis and began using a suction unit and portable respirator. By ten months, he ate only through his epigastric tube (PEG). He became more and more reliant on a suction machine and portable respirator. His secretions got thicker by the day and his voice weaker. At 12 months, he sustained a fall, fracturing a cervical vertebrae, and died from a pulmonary embolism.

Uncle Don and I lived in different cities, so my visits during this period were sporadic, but phone calls were frequent. My uncle joined a nearby out-patient program in an acute care hospital. An occupational therapist taught him to use energy conservation techniques so he could use gravity and leverage to compensate for his weak shoulder muscles. He learned to put his shirt on alone again. His trouser zipper was adapted with a loop so he could close the fly of his pants with greater ease. While he still had some vocal cord motion, the occupational therapist, in conjunction with the speech therapist, taught him forced exhalation exercises to maximize the strength in his vocal cords and prevent aspiration. They also suggested he eat warm (rather than hot or cold) foods, which facilitated his swallowing. They helped him adapt his eating behavior so he could concentrate on eating and limit distraction from human and nonhuman environments. This enhanced his concentration. They taught him and his wife to use the suction machine and respirator.

The occupational therapist gave Uncle Don a few items of adapted equipment, which at first seemed easy to use. He gained control with these gadgets and would readily demonstrate their use. He mastered these techniques and learned a skill which would become essential as the degenerative neurological disease progressed. This enhanced his self-esteem and control over his environment. It worked for him, and it worked for our family.

The second situation involves a friend named Jack. Jack has polio. We have a mutual friend who keeps me posted on his progress. The friend and I are both occupational therapists, but Jack goes to another occupational therapist for treatment—actually he has had many occupational therapists over the decades.

Jack was 25 in 1954 when he contracted polio. He was in law school and married, with a child on the way. Jack was initially placed in an acute care city hospital in an iron lung. Then he was transferred to Boston to a specialty hospital. Finally he was transferred back to New York City, to a long-term care facility. He lived there for fourteen years. He had many losses to cope with: his wife left him and took the child he never saw; he was quadriplegic, and he had to drop out of law school.

After being removed from the iron lung, Jack used a respirator. In time, he learned to "Frog Breathe," or swallow air to force vocalization. He was weaned from the respirator and began to use it only to sleep at night.

Jack had minimal hand function and no gross motor function. His occupational therapists positioned him in an electric wheelchair with a special seat cushion and lapboard. The control for the wheelchair was strategically mounted on the lapboard so he could drive the chair with his wrist, using a joystick. The occupational therapist also designed, fabricated, and modified mouth sticks until she had the best design for Jack. He developed control and strength by hypertrophying his oral musculature.

He learned to operate a computer with his mouth stick. He entered a prevocational training program and learned computer programming, then learned to feed himself, using a balanced forearm orthosis (BFO). Five years ago, after a bout of pneumonia, Jack began using the respirator twice daily in addition to using it at night. He has fractured his right thumb twice and his right hip once. Post-polio syndrome has increased his weakness and fatigue. He uses the respirator more often, at least twice during each meal.

Despite the ups and downs, Jack continues to live a vital life. He works every day. He travels. He has healthy meaningful relationships, including intimate relationships with women.

Jack paces himself, using his time to the fullest. He has attendants who help with his self-care. He sometimes chooses to have help with his ADLs so he can conserve energy for the activities he cherishes the most. He is a prince at balancing work with play.

His occupational therapists have given him advice and helped with necessary adaptations over the years, but he is his own person and controls all aspects of living. Jack lives life to the fullest, in full view of both the obstacles and the rewards.

REFERENCES

Hadley, Linda, "Ventilator-Dependent Patients Gain Freedom with Home Care," *Advance for Occupational Therapists* 3/2/87, pp. 3–5.

Scott, Francie, "Sex and the CORD Patient," *Advance for Occupational Therapists* 1/29/90, p. 12.

Scott, Francie, and E.J. Brown, "Tech-Dependent Kids Become Real Members of the Community," *Advance for Occupational Therapist* 2/26/90, pp. 16–17.

Weitz, Jody, "Mouthstick Enables Young Patient to Excel: O.T.s Determination Pays Off," *Advance for Occupational Therapists* 5(14), p. 5.

31

GOING HOME ON A VENTILATOR

A Nursing Model

Kathleen J. Dunleavy

As early as 1987, it became apparent to the nursing department at Columbia-Presbyterian Medical Center that the option of home ventilation for patients was emerging. It was also evident that planning for such a complex feat would require a master plan.

Under the direction of Susan Bowar-Ferres, R.N., Ph.D., the director of the department, a multidisciplinary task force was formed to study the needs of ventilated patients and plan the teaching required for home ventilation. The task force met for one year, developing and refining protocols and guidelines appropriate to the home-ventilated patient's care. The task force included neuroscience nurses and nursing managers, a neurologist, a pulmonologist, and representatives of the social work services as primary participants.

MASTER PLAN ELEMENTS

This article will describe the elements included in the master plan:

- Selection of patients
- Multidisciplinary team composition
- Teaching protocols/preparations for home
- Supply lists
- Miscellaneous issues/considerations
- Master plan worksheet

SELECTION OF PATIENTS

Selection criteria included the following:

- The patient is stable
- The illness is chronic, not acute
- The patient has a strong desire to be at home
- The patient is able to cope
- The immediate family is able to cope
- A family member is willing to learn requisite care
- Environmental support is adequate
- Financial/insurance support is in place
- An adequate number/type of caregivers is available
- Support systems are in place
- The provisions for medical follow-up are feasible

The decision to be at home is the patient's choice within feasibility parameters. The most common diagnosis of the patients discharged to home is Amyotrophic Lateral Sclerosis (ALS). Although an ALS patient may indicate early in the illness that he or she does not wish to have artificial ventilation, at the time of system/respiratory failure the opinion of the patient may change, and the patient may opt for ventilatory support to relieve the feeling of suffocation. Patients with end stage Multiple Sclerosis (MS) may also opt for home ventilation. One patient who was sent home, who had polymyositis, spent 11 happy months at home with her family before she died.

MULTIDISCIPLINARY TEAM COMPOSITION

To ensure the success of the program, a wide variety of people are actively involved, including:

- Neurology physician
- Pulmonary physician
- Registered nurse(s)
- Social worker
- Respiratory therapist
- Nutritionist, registered dietitian
- Physical therapist
- Home care agency representative
- Utility company representative
- Pastoral care minister
- Patient
- Patient's family members

If required, we also may include utilization review nurses, an occupational therapist, and hospital discharge-planning specialists.

It cannot be stressed enough how vital the organization of the comprehensive team is. Only with all disciplines involved can such a complex mission succeed.

TEACHING PROTOCOLS/PREPARATION FOR HOME

Nursing protocols were divided into two categories: mechanical ventilation and airway management.

The mechanical ventilation protocol included the mechanics of machine functioning, supplies needed, power source needed, alternate power source, oxygen source, equipment, use of equipment, assessing ventilator functioning, troubleshooting machine, travel recommendations, measures used for obstruction or ventilator dysfunction, need for manual ventilating (use of the manual resuscitation bag), contacting emergency services, and the protocol for performing CPR if indicated.

The airway management protocol included respiratory anatomy, mechanics and management of cuffed tracheostomy tube, supplies, tracheostomy care, arrangements for changing tracheostomy tubes, suction machine, suctioning via tracheostomy and orally, and pulmonary toileting. (Chest P.T. as with all patients with restricted mobility.) (As of 1993, the format of the protocols was changed to Marker standards format, but the content remains the same.)

With the help of clear protocols, each step of the teaching is carried out by staff nurses who initial these steps (demonstration, return-demonstration) as more competencies are demonstrated by the family member who has agreed to assume responsibility for the home care needs of the patient. It is essential that at least one family member be trained in the patient's care in the event that a caregiver (usually an LPN) from the home care agency fails to arrive.

Other meaningful educational needs are addressed as necessary (e.g., gastrostomy feedings, care of the gastrostomy—in most cases, feedings are given in boluses as opposed to the hospital procedure of continuous drip for enteral feedings). Basic nursing care (skin care, range of motion, repositioning, oral hygiene, medication administration) is also taught to the appropriate family member.

SUPPLY LIST

A prepared supply list is given to the patient's family when the patient leaves the hospital, and appropriate arrangements are made for the provision and replenishment of these items. The list was generated with input from all members of the team, particularly the staff nurses who do the care and teaching (the real experts).

SPECIAL CONSIDERATIONS

There are many issues present that need to be considered:

1. *Primary Activist.* Implementation of the plan requires at least one discipline to take the lead and coordinate the team's efforts. Initially, nursing was that discipline. Now it can be nursing, the primary physician, the social worker, or all these disciplines. At any rate, the nursing staff conducts approximately 60 percent of the teaching. Nurses schedule and carry out the teaching sessions with the patient and responsible other. The ventilator vendor or respiratory therapist provides the bulk of the mechanical training.

2. *Control Issues.* It is often crucial to a patient's sense of security that he or she feel "in control" of the plan as it evolves. This is achieved by including the patient in all steps of the process and fostering a sense of calmness and normalcy whenever possible.

3. *Simplicity.* Every effort is made to keep the teaching and preparations as clear and simple as possible, to make the plan comfortable for everyone involved. Intensity has no place in the evolution of the plan.

4. *Bonding.* It is essential that the patient develop a sense of trust with the primary players in the plan, particularly with the respiratory therapist who will go home with the patient. In the first home plans developed, we had the services of an unusually caring therapist from the vendor company, who cultivated a wonderful relationship with the patients and personally escorted them home. Today, the respiratory therapist still plays a vital role in the plan, initially by helping the patient and family adjust to the ventilator to be used at home and, importantly, accompanying the patient home and assisting with adjustments at home. Again, every effort is made to keep the process as low-keyed as possible so as to enhance the patient's comfort and trust.

5. *Preparatory Meetings.* A minimum of two meetings were necessary in the first years of home ventilation so that all disciplines could coordinate efforts and troubleshoot problems. As time went on and experience grew, the final "Launching Meeting" became the only necessary interdisciplinary meeting. This meeting enables the team to discuss the outcome of each of their roles and detect any problems or deficiencies. (For the discharge of one end-stage MS patient, even New York's utility company sent a representative to our final "Launching Meeting.")

6. *Agency Caregivers.* Professional caregivers must be in place, with alternate arrangements, should a scheduled caregiver fail to arrive. (The caregivers are usually LPNs). It has been found not only helpful but crucial for caregivers to spend time at the hospital getting to know the patient and

becoming familiar with his or her care. (The registered professional staff nurse teaches the caregivers.)

7. *Care of the Family Caregiver.* It is important that the family have provisions for "respite care" in place. As Moss, Casey, Stocking, et al. said in a recent article on ventilation for ALS patients, ". . . data suggest that home ventilation poses major burdens on family members." Family members need to take care of themselves when the patient resides at home.

8. *Costs.* A home plan is an expensive plan, but cheaper than a hospital stay in most cases. It is said that a home plan can range anywhere from $2,500 to $35,000 a month. Today, a bed alone can cost a patient over $30,000 a month in a hospital.

MASTER PLAN WORKSHEET

A two-page master plan worksheet is used so all disciplines can sign off their readiness and the completion of preparations. The nurse fills in the section related to the completion of the teaching, as do all other disciplines. When each discipline has signed off on its preparations, the patient is ready to be "launched."

SUMMARY

In conclusion, a home plan for the ventilator-dependent patient is a wonderful option for patients under certain circumstances. The plan can result in a happier existence, if it is what the patient wishes. A home plan is complex and costly (yet cheaper than continued hospitalization). A written master plan incorporating all elements of the program can be a helpful tool in implementing a discharge plan.

32

TECHNOLOGICALLY DEPENDENT CHILDREN

Their Effect on the Hospital System

James C. Bernier, M.S.W.
Sarah J. Gossler, M.S.W.

Technologically dependent children represent a growing number of the disabled population. As a group, they raise unique problems for the professionals who care for them. The problems, if unaddressed, may lead to a breakdown in the hospital system. Social workers have a role in helping to maintain the system's functioning.

Traditionally, hospitals have been organized to treat sick individuals, promote health, or provide comfort to terminally ill patients. New technology has stretched the frontiers of the life sciences, particularly with regard to infants and children. The advent of the respirator, new surgical techniques and medications have given new hope to children and their families. Improvements in the care of premature infants, for example, have led to an increase in the number of these children who survive the neonatal period. In 1961, the mortality rate for newborns weighing 1,000 to 1,500 grams (approximately 2-3 pounds) was 50 percent; by the early 1980s it had dropped to 20 percent (President's Commission, 1983). Of infants weighing less than 1,000 grams at birth, half now survive, as compared to 10 percent in the early 1960s.

For most of these neonates, the outlook is good, but not all do well. Some suffer impairments as a result of crises during treatment. Very premature infants may develop a variety of severe chronic life-threatening conditions. In addition, there are significant numbers of children born with congenital anomalies who would not have survived a few years ago. Many of these medically complex infants require frequent hospitalization and intensive medical assistance after their initial discharge from the hospital.

As a result, a new group of children, highly dependent on technological assistance to sustain basic life processes, has been created. Increasingly, infants and children are sent home on respirators. Others are sent home with suctioning machines, apnea monitors, and a host of other services and equipment that in the past would have been provided in a skilled nursing facility (Bock, 1985; Burr, 1983).

These severely impaired children have raised many ethical questions, among them: What relevance does quality of life have in decision making? What burdens do the chronically ill and technologically dependent individual place upon the family in society? What responsibilities do hospital personnel have toward the children and their families, and how is the cost to society balanced against the rights of the individual? Does a child's family have the right to say, at some point, the child's life is no longer worth saving? Does society have the right to dictate whether a child should be saved? In several cases (Clark, Gosnell, and Shapiro, 1981; Press, 1983), the issues have led to sharp debate and intense public scrutiny. This attention has heightened the pressure on the health-care system and necessitated a careful inspection of the civil rights and moral issues involved.

The philosophical and ethical complexities have been examined elsewhere (Fost, 1981). This chapter will explore several stresses these highly charged issues place on the hospital and its staff, who often become quite attached to these children as they deal with them over successive and sometimes prolonged hospitalizations. It will also briefly explore the social worker's role.

DEFINING THE HOSPITAL SYSTEM AND THE SOCIAL WORKER'S ROLE

To consider the impact that technologically dependent patients have on staff, we must look at the larger ecological matrix: the hospital environment. In this context, the institution, the patient, the family, and the community make up one system, with the patient as the focal point. When the organization is functioning at its best, the patient and family seem to be the only system that needs care. The roles of the nurses, physicians, social workers, and other health-care professionals are clearly defined and consensually validated, and there is general agreement on the course of hospitalization. Patients are hospitalized for a specific reason, medical assessment and intervention are provided, and the patient, when able, is discharged. Under these conditions, the hospital personnel can accommodate the individual differences of all members and take care of minor system imbalances.

A social worker's role in these circumstances will be relatively well-defined, depending on how it is prescribed by the institution. The social worker may be called upon to provide discharge planning, procure necessary outpatient services, offer a family emotional support and counseling, or mediate problems between the family and the hospital. Certain crises, such as the impending death of a child, can be unsettling to the hospital, family, and social worker, but these can be resolved and homeostatic balance maintained because the territory is relatively well known. However, medically complex cases raise new questions and require new roles for the social worker. Often, there is a system breakdown, because individuals within the system are called upon to perform in ways which are contrary to tradition. In effect, the hospital needs social work intervention.

WHY AND HOW DOES THE SYSTEM BREAK DOWN?

Since a hospital's basic mission is to cure, technologically dependent children create special problems. Hospitals are action oriented. Hospital staff feels good when it makes someone well, and implicitly views this as its primary function. "A world view that primarily involves sick people who get better may not leave room for the chronically ill or incurable patient, whose defect cannot be fixed" (Darling, 1977). The prognostic and even diagnostic ambiguity of technologically dependent children is a significant stressor on professionals in a treatment-oriented system where results are important. Rosalyn Benjamin Darling quotes a study that found that when doctors were asked which aspects of their careers they found most satisfying, they usually noted "good therapeutic results or a large percentage of successful cases" (Darling, 1977). Since a successful outcome is highly unlikely in these cases, staff is often left with a sense of not knowing what to do, or a feeling that it is not doing the right thing when it may be providing the only treatment possible.

Besides presenting these obstacles, technology dependent children often are developmentally disabled and nonverbal, and cannot make decisions for themselves. Professionals, therefore, must imagine what a child would want, if the child truly understood his or her own needs. Consciously or not, they project themselves into the child's situation by fantasizing how they would feel in facing the degree of helplessness and illness of the child, or they picture themselves as the child's parents.

Even if professionals do not identify with the patient or the parents, they still may question the worth of such a child's life. At some level, each person involved in the care of a technologically dependent child is required to assess how he or she feels regarding prolonging the child's life or hastening death. Leaving it to others may appear to be an easy answer, but the nature of the patient compels each person to assess his or her values. Even those who do not share decision-making powers must decide how aggressively they will attend to their part in the patient's care or how they will relate to the family. For example, nurses required to perform uncomfortable procedures may act less aggressively if they are ethically at odds with the treatment. It seems that "repeated participation [in these moral and ethical dilemmas] does not appear to reduce the worry of the staff about the awesome nature of the decisions" (Duff and Campbell, 1973).

The fundamental issues regarding a dependent population elicit differences in values and individual emotional reactions that tend to polarize staff. Among the social work staff alone, we have witnessed social workers who feel that a retarded patient has a significantly reduced quality of life and should be allowed to die. It is unlikely that this dynamic would not weigh in the manner in which the social worker counsels parents, despite an ethical commitment to the right of self-determination. On the other hand, some social workers agree with physicians who are extremely aggressive in their treatment, arguing that each child has a right to life. They feel that since the child cannot express himself or herself, they must support aggressive life support or honor parents' wish to do so, because they must presume the child wants to live. At times, particularly in cases which are ambiguous and teleologically uncertain, factions can develop and divisions occur between the involved parties. The emergence of these conflicts is often subtle and goes unrecognized at first. Once realized, the problems are not always addressed, because their source lies outside the range of normal staff interactions. Such divisions can affect staff relationships or an individual staff member's psychological adjustment. Despite the importance of these philosophical issues, we have found that interruption of the normal processes of attachment and grief are often more central. These need to be treated in order to keep the organization working smoothly and reduce personal and systemic conflict.

ATTACHMENT AND GRIEF

When considering the impact of the technologically dependent child upon the hospital system, the nature of the staff's attachment to the child needs to be addressed. Because of numerous or prolonged hospitalizations, caretakers frequently develop strong attachments to the children. A child's extreme dependency and need evoke maternal/paternal feelings, particularly among those who provide regular physical and emotional care. The attachment has positive and negative aspects. On the positive side, a loving relationship helps a child grow and develop. Such attachment helps ensure a high level of care, as the staff is more personally invested. Yet there are negative effects. Attachment adds a powerful and complicating dimension to the differences in approach to treatment, value conflicts, questions regarding the quality of life, and the staff's interpersonal relationships, especially when the effect of bonding is unrecognized. The feelings are sometimes unacknowledged because of fear, personal vulnerability, or concern that they might reveal an unprofessional attitude. When unacknowledged, they cannot be dealt with openly, though they are of prime importance. The strong emotions mean that staff often must deal with the added feelings of loss, separation, and grief as a child undergoes a sequence of discharges, admissions, and acute life-threatening episodes. Further, the nature of the child's illness and prognosis interferes with the normal grieving process. At times, the dynamics of the workplace can resemble a family experiencing a complicated grief response as the system seeks to establish homeostasis but is thwarted because it is uncertain whether the child will live or die.

THE COST OF UNCERTAINTY AND PERSONAL ATTACHMENT

The course of life of severely disabled children often cannot be anticipated. Frequent hospitalizations, numerous invasive procedures or crises lead to fluctuating expectations and predictions regarding the final outcome. This chronic contradictory course has an impact on the staff that is not well documented in the literature. We hypothesize that, because of incompletely expressed attachment and grieving issues, the coping process and interpersonal conflicts become further complicated.

Consequently, at any time, a staff member may experience grief, sadness, rage, apathy, or helplessness. Feelings can change from day to day, depending on the child's condition or other factors. Personnel may feel a sense of loss when a child's status changes for the worst or upon admission to or discharge from the hospital. Such vulnerability is usually unexpected by professionals. They may be caught between the hope the child will survive and the desire to see a child's suffering end. Frustration over a particular course of treatment and feelings of helplessness because there is no cure or hope of rehabilitation may lead to feelings of impotence. Coping with the fact that there are no answers, only more uncertainty, is difficult as staff and family members continually prepare for the child to die, only to have him or her survive. This pattern of hope and interrupted grieving is extremely stressful.

Unfortunately, as in the case of attachment, the emotions are often not recognized or acknowledged. Problems arise because the issues may remain submerged yet continue to be played out in daily activities. When this occurs, the system exhibits maladaptive behavior as the staff makes unsuccessful attempts to cope with powerful dynamics and experiences for which it is often unprepared. The reactions come to resemble a pathological grieving process.

SYMPTOMS OF A PATHOLOGICAL COMMUNITY GRIEVING PROCESS

Staff members unable to recognize their own emotional conflicts may become obsessed with the specifics of a child's care, such as blood pressure or changes in temperature, but seem detached when responding to the child's emotional well-being. This detachment may be a defense against past losses or an avoidance of strong feelings of ambivalence. Staff members may express the hope that they are not assigned the care of a particular child. Others become protective or possessive and find themselves in conflict with families and thus experience a type of role confusion. Intense affect, frustration, and anger may be observed. Critical statements regarding other members of the team, which may take the form of blaming, are also symptoms of this uncertainty. Passive/aggressive behavior among an otherwise well-functioning group, urgent referrals to yet another specialty to "do something," or feelings of worthlessness and doubt regarding one's own and other professionals' competence should alert the social worker to these unspoken undercurrents.

Staff Relationship With Parents

While the staff is adapting to the above issues, it must not be forgotten that the parents are also having problems with thwarted expectations, guilt, and attachment. Solnit and Start (1961) first documented the problems parents of handicapped children must face as they grieve the loss of the wished-for child and grow to love the child they have been given. The loss remains a poignant reality and, as Gath (1985) suggests, "the very success of family planning has meant that each child is planned to be perfect, embodying more of the parental aspirations than a generation or two ago, when many families could expect to lose a child through early death." The uncertainty that technologically dependent youngsters bring necessarily exacerbates the grief process, because even basic nurturant behavior can sometimes precipitate a crisis (Gath, 1985). Imagine how a mother feels when her child, who has severe swallowing difficulties, must be hospitalized with pneumonia following the aspiration of food. Parent and baby cannot engage in the usually pleasurable and highly reinforcing act of feeding. Sleep is not a time of rest and recuperation for a parent whose child has apnea and must be on a monitor. These and similar issues effect the daily lives of parents and child.

Drotar, et al. (1975) described the reluctance parents of a congenitally malformed children feel in becoming attached to their babies who might die. Eventually, these parents reorganize and adapt, but "the recurrent hospitalizations required for the care of many children with malformations intensified parental anxieties, which had been initially created by the babies' births and might start the process of reactions over again." At times their reactions resemble acute grief reactions, exhibiting renewed denial, guilt, somatic complaints, agitation, disorganization, and distorted reactions (Lindemann, 1944). It is no wonder that parents faced with such stress react in atypical ways when a child is hospitalized.

Because of extended periods of medical care, staff becomes familiar with these parents, their shortcomings, psychological symptoms, and the stresses they endure. While on the one hand they can be very supportive and emotionally connected with the families, conflicts may emerge as the systemic boundaries and roles become ill-defined. These families experience a wide range of emotions, including anger and frustration, that they may direct toward themselves, the child, or health-care professionals (Drotar, et al., 1975; Vachon, 1979).

Though personnel may be intellectually aware that family members are displacing the anger resulting from their feelings of helplessness, they may react in nonrational ways because of their own internal conflicts. Professionals may come to see the family disorganization not as a symptom of stress, but as a cause of the child's problems or something the family deserves by virtue of their behavior or social status.

Even though all parties wish to do what is right, feelings of impotence and the inability to affect change sometimes lead to mutual blame. Staff and parents may become polarized, each seeing the other as an element in the child's lack of progress. It is less threatening to accuse someone of being inadequate than it is to deal with personal problems and resolve differences. It is easier, and sometimes safer, for a parent to be angry at a nurse than to be angry at a spouse who seems not to care enough to bring a child home on a respirator. It is easier for a nurse or doctor to blame a parent for not giving a sick child a home than to deal with the fact that there is simply no change. It is easier to see parents as having unrealistic expectations than to risk hoping a child may improve or survive with a significantly reduced quality of life. When the best interest of the child is an open question or people cannot decide what is morally right, it is easier to place the responsibility on others. Both the parents and the staff deal with grieving and uncertainty by displaying anger, feelings of impatience, and wishes to escape the responsibilities raised.

Control—Whose Child Is This, Anyway?

When both staff and parents are emotionally invested in a child whose existence awakens conflict, the issue of control is central to the way stress is handled. One mother posed the question this way, "Whose child is this, anyway?"

Who decides whether life is worth living in the face of such ambiguity? Can parents refuse to follow medical advice, or can the medical establishment refuse to follow the wishes of parents? Can someone care and yet leave the crucial decisions to someone else? Dealing with families of technologically dependant children is a significant stressor for the hospital system. The staff struggles with its own attachment to both the family and the child, with its own conflicts, hopes, and expectations.

Communication Breakdown Due to Fragmentation of Case

Finally, while there is only one family, which forms a whole and relatively unchanging system, the medical setting is composed of many people who are often loosely connected. A nurse on one shift, who is working part-time, does not have the benefit of interaction with other nurses and may convey entirely different messages or expectations to family members. A parent who visits evenings cannot know how the day shift feels, and yet it directs the course of the care and formulates policy. Feeling isolated, the staff does not benefit from seeing that everyone is struggling. It wonders whether anyone cares, simply because of the lack of opportunity to explore its feelings.

THE SOCIAL WORKER'S ROLE

As professionals knowledgeable in psychodynamics and systems theories, social workers are in a unique position to intervene therapeutically when the system is malfunctioning. They can educate the hospital staff about the process of community grieving and how it manifests itself. In doing so, the social worker can raise awareness and help clarify values and emotional issues by focusing on the complex factors involved in the care of these children. He or she can help fellow professionals acknowledge their ambivalence and the problems that grow out of uncertainty surrounding the prognosis. When skillfully done, these efforts are usually welcomed. Sometimes, simply making appropriate observations enables those involved to come to terms with the issues involved.

If a social worker has an opportunity to participate in support meetings or nursing or pediatric rounds, it is possible to address systemic problems during these sessions. These forums provide an excellent opportunity to foster the staff's understanding of the issues of grief and its feelings of isolation and frustration. Often the social worker may wish to act as the family's representative at these meetings, since the family is usually not present and feelings can be projected or displaced onto them. By representing the family, the social worker not only can prevent scapegoating but also can bring the issues of grieving and attachment into focus.

Although participation in regular ongoing support meetings is the ideal, it is more likely that cases will have to be dealt with on an individual basis. The following is an example drawn from our clinical experience. While it does not contain all the elements discussed thus far, it is an example of system breakdown and successful mediation.

THE CASE OF SOK MAO

S was a four-year-old Cambodian child who was severely retarded. For the first three years of her life, her treatment had been characterized by long hospital stays, with brief trips home. Over the next two years, the situation gradually changed. By the time she was four, she spent nearly all her time at home but also had frequent stays in the hospital.

During her first three years, S was frequently connected to a ventilator. Because she was intubated so often, it was decided to perform a tracheostomy, and this resulted in some improvement in her condition. A gastrostomy tube was also inserted into her stomach, enabling her to be fed without aspirating her food, thus solving a problem she had with frequent aspiration pneumonias. She was sent home with the gastrostomy tube and the tracheostomy, which required frequent suctioning. In addition, she needed a cardiac monitor and an oxygen mist tent.

S did well and, over time, it was felt sufficient progress had been made and the tracheostomy was closed. However, following closure, respiratory distress gradually began to develop. It was determined that not enough air was getting through under normal breathing conditions and that another tracheostomy needed to be performed.

When permission was requested to operate again, the parents refused. A social worker was called, ostensibly because a referral to the child protective agency would need to be made if the parents declined to permit the operation.

In exploring the issues, the social worker found that both direct care staff, especially the nurses, and physicians had requested the consult, but each referred with different intentions. To the referring physician, the problem was the parents' refusal to give surgical consent and the need to engage the authorities. For the nurses, the focus was slightly different. They had spent many months nurturing S and had grown quite attached. To some, the parents seemed to be requesting euthanasia and were seen as cold and rejecting. They made statements regarding what was presumed to be an ethnic tendency not to value developmentally delayed children. To others, the parents' attitude was seen as merciful. However, the staff showed no recognition of its own deep attachment to a child it had seen through many crises over the years. What emerged was a pattern of blame shifting, covert alliances that were acted out in various ways.

The parents, on their part, were not asking for assistance. The social worker was seen in the role of enforcer. The mother and father revealed to the social worker that when they consented to the first tracheostomy, they believed the operation would eventually restore their child to normalcy. They had given her excellent care and loved their child deeply; however, they felt S wanted to be left alone.

After performing an initial assessment, the social worker identified the focus of intervention as the medical and family system interface. It was evident there were unacknowledged attachments, miscommunication, cultural differences, a variety of value systems, and other issues that needed to be addressed. A meeting was called between the physician, key floor staff, the parents, and the social worker.

Using standard interviewing and intervention techniques, the social worker was able to elicit the parents' true compassion and concern, as well as demonstrate the physical investment they had made in the child. This allowed the staff to see them in a different perspective.

The nurses were able to validate the parents' concerns and the validity of their viewpoint. Those who felt threatened by the loss were permitted to express their fears, while seeing that they were not alone in thinking of S's benefit. The physician was then able to explain his predicament of not having any choice but to pursue surgery because of legal dilemmas. In explaining their own concerns, the nurses came to realize their own attachment and thereby saw the parents' decision in a different light. The parents came to appreciate the deep level of caring that the nurses and physicians had for S. As a result, all were able to agree to pursue surgery, feeling united in their concern for the child, and to see themselves struggling with the ambiguities of the situation.

CONCLUSION

Technologically dependent children represent a growing number of the disabled population. As a group, they raise unique problems for the professionals who care for them. Some of these difficulties, such as the moral and ethical problems regarding quality of life and the avoidance of unnecessary, painful treatment, have provoked much professional discussion and have received a good deal of attention in the popular press. Other issues have received relatively little explanation. The cultural, psychological, and emotional needs of those involved in the child's care, if left unacknowledged or unresolved, often lead to a breakdown in the health-care system. Social workers, because of their unique perspective, have a role in helping to maintain the system's functioning. They can bring their expertise to bear in a therapeutic way by educating the system, helping clarify values and emotional issues, and helping everyone to deal with a complex grieving process.

REFERENCES

Brock, R.H., "State of the Art: Pediatric Home Care in 1985," *Caring* 1985,IV(5): 26–28.

Burr, B.H., B. Guyer, I.D. Todres, et al., "Home Care for Children on Respirators," *New England Journal of Medicine* 1983, 309: 1319–1323.

Clark, M., M. Gosnell, and D. Shapiro, "When Doctors Play God," *Newsweek* (August 31, 1981), pp. 48–54.

Darling, R.B.,"Parents, Physicians, and Spina Bifida," *Hastings Center Report* (August 1977), 7(5): 10–14.

Drotar, D., B.A. Paskiewicz, N. Irvin, J. Kennell, and M. Klaus, "The Adaption to the Birth of an Infant with a Congenital Malformation: A Hypothetical Model," *Pediatrics* 1975, 56: 710–717.

Duff, R.S., and M.B. Campbell, "Moral and Ethical Dilemmas in the Special Care Nursery, *New England Journal of Medicine* 1973, 289(17): 890–894.

Fost, N., "Ethical Issues in the Treatment of Critically Ill Newborns," *Pediatric Annals* 1981, 10(10): 383–389.

Gath, A., "Parental Reactions to Loss and Disappointment: The Diagnosis of Down Syndrome," *Developmental Medicine and Child Neurology* 1985, 27: 392–400.

Lindemann, E., "Symptomatology and Management of Acute Grief," *The American Journal of Psychiatry* 1944, 101: 15–18.

President's Commission for the Study of Ethical Problems in Medicine, Biomedical and Behavioral Research, Seriously Ill Newborns (March 1983), "Deciding to Forego Life Sustaining Treatment: A Report on the Ethical, Medical, and Legal Issues in Treatment Decisions," pp. 197–229.

Press, J.E., "The Story of Baby Doe," *New England Journal of Medicine* 1983, 309: 64.

Solnit A.J., and M.H. Start, "Mourning the Birth of a Defective Child," *Psychoanalytic Study of Child* 1961, 6: 523–537.

Vachon, M.L.S., "Staff Stress in Care of the Terminally Ill," *QRB/Quality Review Bulletin* May 1979: 13–17.